The Art and Knowledge of
Thai Yoga Massage

To my family

The Art and Knowledge of Thai Yoga Massage

Attila Pegán

Licensed Masage Therapist (LMT);
Practitioner and Instructor;
Savage, Minnesota

 Humania KnowledgeBase

Attila Pegan

12629 Natchez ave. Savage, MN 55378

aboutfaceyourbody@hotmail.com

The Art and Knowledge of Thai Yoga Massage   ISBN: 978-963-06-8869-7

First Edition

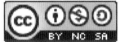
Note

The author will not be liable for any loss or damage of any nature occasioned to or suffered by any persons arising out of or related to any use of the material contained in this book.

Contents

Preface

Since Asokananda's original book series, The Art of Traditional Thai Massage, many books and educational materials have been published to share and spread the healing tradition of ancient Thailand. In the last 30 years, the activities of numerous practitioners, receivers, authors and supporters of Thai massage have powered a movement that we can easily call the renaissance of Thai Massage. It is becoming more popular than ever, practiced around the globe. The Thai Massage movement can help bring back the preventive principle of medicine, making us more resilient and better able to reach our goals by keeping us healthier and more productive in our lives.

This growing popularity of Thai massage in the western world has yielded the possibility for this book to be published. What began as a workshop handout for beginning practitioners has grown beyond all my expectations during 2 years of development. It has become not just a textbook but a platform for the practice, research and organization of the Thai massage community.

This textbook will guide practitioners who want to add Thai massage to their existing practice modalities, as well as those who are considering making Thai massage the cornerstone of their practice. The former will find satisfaction by adding different perspective and effective techniques to their existing practice, while the latter will take the practice to the next level of healing and craftsmanship.

The work and research that led to the publishing of this textbook is in its early stage. After the rediscovery, and subsequent differentiation of Thai massage from Western knowledge and practices, we now move toward integration. During this phase of the work I am focusing on including and carrying on all substantial elements to aid in the process of integrating different views, traditions and practices.

It is my hope that many of you who are taking the spiritual journey that is Thai massage will some day travel to Thailand and immerse yourself in the culture that carried on this healing art.

Minnesota, 2009   Attila Pegán

Acknowledgements

I have started this project by my self and during the course of the development of this book many bright minded people helped, formed and influenced the work and the final outcome. I would like to thank them and send them a respectful bow to make this book as user friendly as it is. To Roz, Bo, Cameron and Gavy for giving me plenty of time and space which might otherwise have been theirs. To Miki who has initiated this work and helping me since with the organization of the material. To Connie for taking on my writings and making good sense of it. To Balázs for being a friend and traveling, studying together from the beginning of our carrier. To Andrea and Laurino for their teachings. To Tom Myers and the faculty of KMI for giving me a new direction in bodywork and in life. To Ma Devi who shared the tradition of yoga with me. To Sunny and Cari the directors of the CenterPoint School for supporting my teachings and running a fantastic school in Minneapolis and to Elizabeth, Melis, Connie, Roz, Lorelle, Sarah Marie, Lori for giving up their bodies for the pictures and recordings.

Introduction

In 1999 I found myself looking to make a career change as I had become tired of IT and working with machines. I sought work that involved people in a more relaxed environment. That summer I attended a conference about sports related recreation. The doctor/manual therapist of the Hungarian Olympic Team caught my attention with a presentation about his work and relationships with the athletes. It inspired me so much that I signed up for a 20 hour relaxation massage course. After the short exam of giving and receiving massage my body was happy and laughing and I knew this is what I wanted to do in my next vocation.

After taking a number of short massage courses with different practitioners I eventually discovered Thai Massage. I took a weekend workshop in Budapest, where I lived at that time, and the next thing I knew I was on an airplane heading to Thailand for more. I stayed for 2 months and studied almost the whole time at the ITM school in Chiang Mai, mostly because back then they were the only school with a website. ITM was a good option for me as I wasn't a yogi or an experienced massage therapist, just a newbie with some knowledge of anatomy, physiology and bodywork who was just learning English.

But the first thing that affected me wasn't the massage; it was the yoga practice every morning before class. After 5 weeks of daily yoga I became able to listen and pay attention to my bodily sensations much clearer. The Thai massage class and practice was so new that my friend Balázs and I practiced every day after class until around 9 pm. We knew that if we wanted to improve in Thai massage, we needed to practice the new moves and stretches right away to feel our bodies in the poses so we could remember the techniques when giving a massage. We only knocked off for the evening when the pancake boy stopped by our house on his route to the night market. We would dine on Muslim fried pancakes, a popular street food filled with banana, chocolate syrup or egg, and topped with sugar.

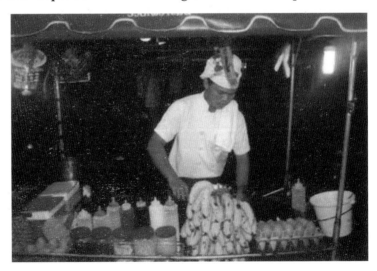

Illustration 1. Pancake boy

The 2 months went fast and soon I was back in Hungary, starting a certification program in medical massage for licensing reasons, but my real interest remained in Thai massage. I finished the program in about 7 months and moved to the USA, and to the home of my new wife, Minnesota. It was quite a challenge to introduce Thai massage to the local community and it deepened my feelings about the superiority of the East over the West. I continued to take advanced Thai massage courses in the U.S. and Canada and eventually I went back to Thailand for training as a teacher's assistant with Andrea in the Lahu Village. This time I spent more time living with Thais and traveling around the country with Roz and our 3 children.

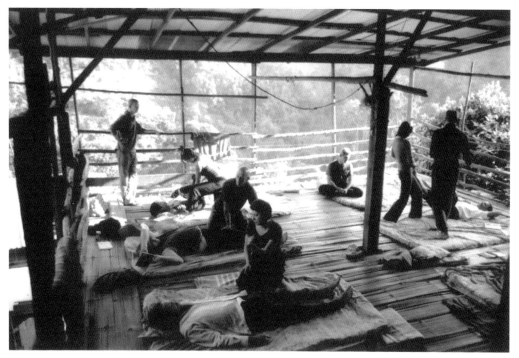

Illustration 2. Thai massage course at the Lahu village - Northern Thailand

One day after getting back to the States I was surfing the web for a massage article and the book cover of Anatomy Trains – an illustration with colorful longitudinal lines laid over Albinus' standing skin-and-adipose-tissue-less model - pulled up on my screen. I didn't know what I was looking at but it was very familiar from my studies of the Sen Energy Lines of Thai massage.

I purchased the book and I read it, and though I didn't completely understand it I felt this was something I was missing. I signed up for the next Anatomy Trains workshop and after attending it I understood. East and West met in me; Thai massage is very intuitive and experience based and Anatomy Trains and its professional training the KMI are very scientific and knowledge base.

My East oriented heart became refreshed and balanced by a heavy load of sensible and living Western applied anatomy. I began researching the Thai Sen Energy Lines and their resemblance to the longitudinal paths and connections of the body wide network of our connective tissue.

This textbook and the DVD, training courses and related activities are designed to aid this research into Traditional Thai massage. Not only to deepen our knowledge and intuition on the way toward its roots, but to increase access to touch for practitioners and receivers alike.
It is a work in progress and I would like to invite you to participate and contribute to it any way you are able.

PART I
THE TRADITION OF THAI MASSAGE

History

Nuad Phaen Boran or Nuad Bo Rarn is the Thai name of Traditional Thai Massage which has over 2500 years of history. While the layperson would think it is originated from Thailand, the truth is that the roots of Thai massage lie not in Thailand but in Northern India, where the legendary founder of Thai massage Jivaka Kumar Bhaccha, an ayurvedic doctor lived.

Jivaka studied medicine for seven years under a famous ayurvedic teacher Punarvasu, who was commonly known as Atreya. Jivaka became one of Aatreya's best students and received the entirety of Atreya's Ayurvedic healing knowledge. One of the written story documents Jivaka's final exam for the graduation from the Taksasila University, Atreya's school. Aatreya told his students to bring back to the classroom all the plants, animal products and minerals that had no medicinal value, from around the medical school's vicinity. The students had a week to accomplish this task and by the end of the week they all came back, laden with baskets and carts full. All but Jivaka, who came back empty-handed. Jivaka then told his teacher, Aatreya, that he realized that everything in nature is filled with healing power. So Jivaka passed the final test and a well known ayurvedic aphorism was created:

"There is no syllable without mantric power; there is no person without good qualities; similarly there is no root [herb] without medicinal power. Rare is the one who can discover these powers and put them to good use.[1]"

Jivaka became the most celebrated doctor in Northern India during the Buddha period, around 500 B.C. His unusual skill as a physician and a surgeon was well known. He was called upon to treat kings and princes, including the king of the empire, Bimbisara. But of all the distinguished people Jivaka treated, his greatest pleasure was to attend to Prince Siddhartha Gautama the Buddha himself, which he did three times a day.

While Jivaka specialized in the healing of the physical body, the Buddhist tradition considers Buddha as the doctor of the mind and his knowledge of the Dharma[2] as the medicine. "He used the knowledge of the Dharma to heal the illness that arose from the three poisons: greed, ager, and ignorance.[3]" Their friendship developed with the time to the point that Buddha handed the medical responsibility for himself and the leadership of his followers to Jivaka. After Buddha's enlightenment and passing, Jivaka went to Tibet and established Buddhist medicine based on their collaboration.

Jivaka's medical teachings and practice -embedded into Theravada Buddhism- spread so well that the Thai culture kept him as one of their religious figures. They called him 'Father of Medicine' by the name of Shivago Komparaj. Today the mantra Om Namo Shivago is chanted daily in most Thai massage schools in his honor.

According to several studies and researches, the influence of Jivaka on Traditional Thai Medicine and Thai Massage is irrefutable, but it is more likely that Thai Massage was forged and influenced by much broader knowledge and sources, even from as far away as Europe, as we'll see below.

During the next centuries Buddhism and its healing practices were spreading through India, within the growing Maurya Empire which stretched from modern Bangladesh on the East to modern Afghanistan on the west and was ruling most of the Indian sub-continent. Asokha the king of the empire converted to Buddhism and sponsored the propagation of Buddhism not only in his empire but outside of India by sending emissaries to foreign countries and territories.

Buddhism then started to spread around the world in every direction. The important direction for us is the East, as beyond Sri Lanka, Bangladesh and Burma, the region of modern Thailand where early trading settlers were forming organized states. Around the 2nd century B.C. Ashoka proselytized the population of these states, amongst them the Mon ethnic group. They are believed to be responsible for the spread of Theravada Buddhism[4] in the region.

The history of this region is mostly unknown before and during the Mon, Khmer and Malay dynasties up until the time of the migrating Tais[5] arrived from the Tokin region of modern Vietnam, through the Chinese province of Yunnan. It is believed that the Buddhist medical practice from India had mixed and melted with Chinese medicine, and the indigenous medicine that was practiced in Siam[6] had also been absorbed, and became the basis of the Traditional Thai medicine.

The first well established state of Thailand was Sukhothai, and later Ayuthaya became the capital of the region. If there was documentation of Thai medicine it most likely was destroyed in 1767 when the Burmese invaders burned and destroyed Siam's old royal capital Ayuthaya. The only remaining complete text is the Tamraa phra osot Phra Narai ("Medical Texts of King Narai")[7] that lead to the reconstruction effort of Thai medicine by order of King Rama III later in the nineteenth century. This work took place at the famous Wat Pho (Wat Phra Chetuphon) temple in Bangkok which became the "democratic university of comprehensive education,"[8] influenced by western ideals. The original documents were etched into marble slabs, and several other statues were also made that resemble yoga and Thai massage poses.

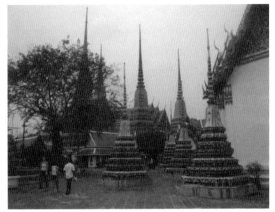

Illustration 3. The garden of the Wat Pho with the pagodas in the back - Bangkok

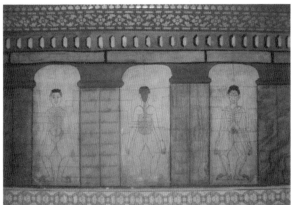

Illustration 4. The famous carvings of the Sen Lines

These remains are somewhat overshadowed by the main attraction of the Wat Pho, the largest side lying Buddha in Thailand or perhaps in the world. The charts and carvings are located in several small, open aired pagodas. Most of them are put up over the head and they are small in size, maybe 3-4 feet tall. Other ones with color paintings are on the walls. Interestingly, some of the drawings are not humans but rather some kind of Gods or fighters with specific energetic points and lines. They look like applications to prepare soldiers for battle, or treatments for the injured ones.

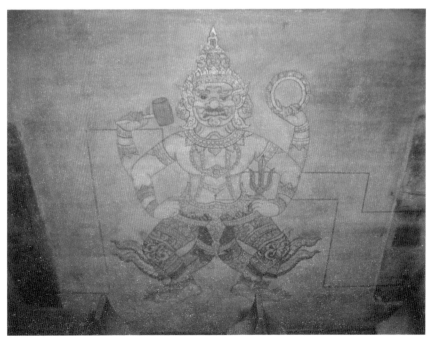

Illustration 5. Painting with reference points of the body

The 24 sculptures in the garden of the temple are posing in different yoga postures. These are representing the „Lu Si Da Ton", the Thai version of Hatha yoga. They call them "contorted hermit positions" and these are the basis of a complex exercise routine that can be done solo or with a partner. These positions are influenced by the Indian yoga tradition.

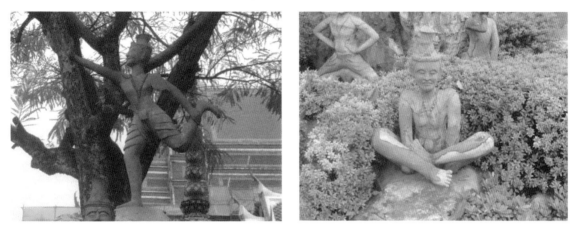

Illustration 6-7. Lu Si Da Ton sculptures in the garden of the Wat Pho

Later in 1907, collections of all the known traditional medicine sources were published: "...the Tamrå phesat ("Texts on Medicine") and the Phåetthayasåt songkhro ("The Study of Medicine"), as well as an abridged version of the above titles for students, the Wetchasuakså phåetthayasåtsangkhap ("Manual for Students of Traditional Medicine")— are still in use by the Wat Pho Traditional Medical College Association for the training of traditional physicians. Courses in traditional medicine across Thailand continue to utilize these texts as the cornerstone of their training programs."[9]

The Wat Pho Temple was and still is the center of the Southern style of Thai massage. This style is known for strong pressure and rather aggressive movements, some of them similar to chiropractic adjustments and rigorous workout-like treatments mostly focusing and working with the nervous system and joints. On the other hand, during the centuries a somewhat lighter, more rhythmic and relaxing Northern style[10] developed in the northern region of the country within the center of the city of Chiang Mai. The two modalities are born of the separation of the kingdom where the king's class ruled the life of the poor agricultural workers. Therefore the king's class had its own style - the southern, specialized for internal organs, nervous system and joint mobilization, while the poor had their local monks and folk healers treating their work-related conditions, focusing on general mobility, leg, hip and back issues.

Traditional Thai massage almost died out in Thailand as western medical interests moved into the country in the last century. Soon hospitals and pharmacies were offering medication, drugs and surgeries and people started to abandon the traditional treatments and practitioners. Thailand became the strategic stronghold and popular destination for the armed forces during the South-East-Asian wars. Young people of the same generation of the 60's and 70's hippy revolution also turned to the ancient east and started to learn about Buddhism, meditation and traveled to Asia. Some of these people rediscovered Thai massage on their quest to enlightenment and stuck around to learn from the local practitioners and started to assemble the knowledge that is available for us today. One of them was Asokananda, a German native who became a Buddhist monk and spent many years recovering our healing art.

History and today's revival of Traditional Thai Medicine clearly show 3 main fields in Traditional Thai Medicine; Thai herbal and dietary therapies, Traditional Thai Massage and body therapies, and spiritual practices (what Salguero calls Magico-religious healing[11]).

As you can see, Thai massage has always been part of a broader, more wholistic approach to healing and medicine. Before we start focusing on Thai massage remember this context and apply it accordingly.

References:
1 For the full story and other Buddhist teachings visit
   http://www.aboutfaceyourbody.com/tiki-index.php?page=BookPage
2 One of the three jewels of Buddhism, means the teaching of Buddha. The other 2 jewels are Buddha and Sangha
3 Buddhism, medicine and health book
4 "the teaching of the Elders", the oldest Buddhist school and tradition known as closest to Buddha's original teachings
5 refers to the ancient ethnic group of that name
   refer to the people of modern Thailand.
6 The official name of Thailand until June 23 1939
7 ,8 Salguero, The History of Traditional Thai Medicine Reconsidered pp. 14
9 Salguero, The History of Traditional Thai Medicine Reconsidered pp. 14
10 For more about the modern history of Thai massage visit
    http://www.aboutfaceyourbody.com/tiki-index.php?page=BookPage
11 Salguero, The History of Traditional Thai Medicine Reconsidered pp. 16

Foundation – The six pillars of Thai massage

The foundation of Thai massage was built and refined throughout the history of Thai medicine. The undeniable link to Iron Age India, the local traditions of indigenous tribes in Siam and the customs of Thai immigrants formed the base of Thai massage, and has been revamped and recollected during a time of growing western and global interest. By tracing these influences, we can identify 6 genuine practices that melted together in Thai massage.

1. Metta

Metta is a Pāli[1] word, that I like to use in English, translated as "loving - kindness" or "active interest in others". Metta is a core piece of Theravāda Buddhism and also a popular form of Buddhist meditation. Metta is a general state of life, an ongoing positive feeling towards people and any living, sentient being. It is love without attachment. Metta lives inand flows from the heart, or 4th, Chakra in the middle of the chest. The exchange and cultivation of Metta is a central spiritual principle and is the main goal of Buddhism and most world religions- as the optimum state of existence. As my friend Eldor says: "Everybody would like to love and to be loved".

In Thai massage, Metta is the fabric of the relationship of practitioner, receiver and the greater community of people involved in our healing art. You can probably see, feel and sense these qualities by working and studying with Thai massage people. If nothing else, the specific and very thoughtful massage treatments stand out. This built-in consciousness, openness and love allows us to tap into the energetic and intuitive levels of practice, and as a result the massage affects not only the giver, the receiver and the immediate environment and surrounding people, but sends a ripple effect throughout the collective unconsciousness and helps to bring a better life for all.

Metta as a foundation of Thai massage gets varying degrees of attention in courses, trainings and sessions. Metta depends on both the practitioner or teacher and the receiver. Openness is needed from both sides, such that I can say that Thai massage is not for everybody. People tend to be reserved.

I discovered Metta later in my practice. At the beginning I didn't hear about it and nobody mentioned it in class. I just noticed in myself a very good feeling while doing, receiving and learning Thai massage. Then at my first training with the Sunshine Network[2] in Montreal, Canada, I was listening to Andrea and Laurino -who are both advanced practitioners of meditation- and we chanted the Om Mani Padme Hum mantra

17

and all of a sudden I could pinpoint Metta –first as a warming feeling in my heart and chest and my whole body and then from the individual attention I received from them- which later became the framework of my practice, the secret ingredient of Thai massage. I came to the conclusion that bringing love into my practice is the most important part of Thai massage.

2. Meditation

Basic meditation is the application of Metta in Thai massage. Additionally, being mindful and focused about what you do in your practice is a form of meditation even if it doesn't include hours of sitting and chanting or going for a silent retreat.

Vipassana[3], for the more adventurous is one of the traditional Buddhist silent meditations that is popular among Thai massage practitioners. It is a universal, scientific method towards purifying the mind, with the standard perspective of "Looking at things and happenings as they are". The goal of this meditation is to live life without cravings and rejection while cultivating a neutral, non-judgmental state of mind. In scientific terms the left and right sides of the brain are processing information from our senses in different ways. The left brain is in a constant state of organization and classification based on our polarized and ambivalent self image. It stamps every piece of information as "good" or "bad", and forces the mind to crave after the good and reject the bad. The right brain processes information in an intuitive way and lets the information flow through the mind.

The Buddha, one of the originators of Vipassana, noticed that every piece of information that reaches the mind triggers a body-wide response in the form of a slight move. These movements can be detected and neutralized with a clear mind and focused attention, and ultimately can derail the deeply imprinted response cycle of the thought process, and can thus liberate and enlighten a person.

This central piece of Vipassana, the heightened attention to bodily sensations, is very useful in the practice of Thai massage. It aids in sensing and understanding the receiver's condition –through your own experience - and will lead to more effective sessions.

Asokananda's Sunshine Network is heavily involved in meditation, so if you are seeking to enhance your Thai massage practice with silent meditation I recommend attending one of their classes or look for a local Vipassana group.

3. Yoga

The yoga tradition is a discipline of mental and physical practices. Its history can be traced back as far as the Indus Valley Civilization (c. 3300-1700 BCE) based on artifacts that depict yoga and meditation-like poses. During the Bronze and Iron Ages in India, Yoga evolved from the mystic practices of the ascetics to become a central component of Hinduism, Buddhism and Jainism. The main source texts of yoga are the Upanishads, (ca. 400 BCE), and the Mahabharata, including the famous Bhagavad Gita (ca. 200 BCE). These texts were collected and compiled by Patanjali in the second century BCE and we know them as the Yoga Sutras of Patanjali.

These Yoga Sutras became the basis of Classical or Ashtanga Yoga. The ultimate goal of Classical Yoga is enlightenment for the eventual liberation from the cycle of birth and death by following the golden middle path through the 8 steps or folds. The 8 steps are Yama, Niyama, Asana, Pranayama, Pratyahara, Dharana, Dhyana, Samadhi. These can be translated as abstentions, observances, seated position, restrain breath, Abstraction, Concentration, Meditation, Liberation.

The central concept of the Yoga tradition is Prana, or vital energy, that we sense and stimulate in Thai Massage. We will pay special attention to the Pranic system in Part III.

4. Hatha Yoga - Stretching and breathing

Hatha yoga is known as a physical exercise practice in the western world. It is actually a portion of the original 8 limbed Classical Yoga Path.

On the 8 folded path the 3rd fold is the Asana and the 4th is Pranayama. Taken together they comprise Hatha yoga. Asana means poses, or movements, and originally Asanas were designed to improve one's ability to remain in a seated position for extended periods of time during meditation. It has since evolved into a series of stretching exercises. Pranayama, the 4th fold, controls the life force or Prana and its manifestation in the breath by teaching techniques of inhalation and exhalation. This combination of physical exercises and breathing techniques greatly influences physical and mental health.

The influence of the Yoga tradition is evident in Thai massage. It is often called lazy men's yoga or assisted yoga and if you look at the exercises such as Cobra, Locust or the Tree pose you will find the exact Hatha yoga poses for the receiver. What is also interesting but somewhat hidden is that the practitioner is doing his or her own Hatha yoga during the Thai yoga massage session. Thai massage exercises often demand greater flexibility and more specific stretches from the practitioner than from the receiver. Also, the synchronizing of movement with the breath during a massage session is essential, just like in a solo Hatha Yoga practice.

5. Movement therapy

One of the beauties of Thai massage is its movement. The synchronous and often mirroring moves during a session enables both practitioner and receiver to get proper physical exercise. For the therapist the work is integrates all the complexities of the body and its weights, angles, leverage and balance points in a highly sensitive and feedback driven environment for the length of the session. With correct body mechanics it helps practitioners stay fit, strong and flexible.

For the receiver it is a different story. The body's basic protocols for sensory and motor nerve function are challenged or even interrupted during Thai massage. The sensory nerve fibers - especially the mechanoreceptors that sense body movement and pressure placed against the body- transmit the signals from movements, pressure, stretches, etc. to the brain for processing, then a signal is sent back to the motor nerves to trigger a movement or an action by electrifying the muscle tissue. During a Thai massage, the receiver is encouraged to let go and relax -as I usually hint: don't move a muscle-to lower or cut off the flow toward the motor neurons. Results of this circumstance are highly beneficial to the receiver's nervous system, and also enable the practitioner to better observe any holding patterns, restricted muscles, muscle groups and areas of the body.

The other well known benefits of Thai massage are looser skeletal muscle tone, greater range of motion and heightened energy level, all of which stem from the movements of the practice.

6. Acupressure

It is the most common technique in Thai massage. It originated from China as part of Traditional Chinese Medicine, where the acupoints of the Chinese meridian system are treated by pressure from the fingers, hands, elbows or mechanical devices.

In Thai massage, acupressure is applied along the Thai Sen Energy lines, which are different from Chinese meridians and acupoints. The flow of energy in the Sen Lines is induced by pressing a certain point or area, or by the rhythmic change of place and location where pressure takes place. The level of expertise of acupressure applied in Thai massage ranges from thumbing and elbow pressure to use of the feet and often sometimes the weight of the practitioner's body on the receiver.

Reflexology is a specific application of acupressure. Pressure is applied over the so-called Micro-areas of the body; the hands, feet, ears and face. These areas represent the entire body and the organs. Specific areas can be affected by pressing them through complex neurological, energy-based and fascial connections. Thai massage has adapted the principles and practice of reflexology as a secondary positive side effect. The main focus is still on stimulating the Sen Lines and the energy flow while the reflex effects from pressure on the Micro-areas are acknowledged. It adapted so well that many Thai massage schools teach Thai reflexology courses by using a small rounded stick to treat internal organ points on the feet.

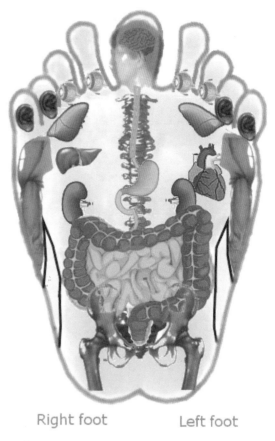

Right foot   Left foot

Illustration 8 - Reflex zones of the feet

References:

1 an Indo-Aryan language used as the liturgical and scholarly language   of Theravada Buddhism. "Pali." Merriam-Webster Online Dictionary. 2009.
2 Visit www.asokananda.com for further information and courses
3 www.vridhamma.org link to the Vipassana Research Institute (VRI) website

Style and techniques

Thai massage is really different from western massage modalities. The most stunning difference is the length of the session. In Thai massage an average full body massage session is about 2 hours long and can easily be longer. In the western world it is quite challenging for most people, not only for receivers but -as I discovered during my teaching- for practitioners too.

Two distinct styles have been developed within Thai massage during the centuries (as already mentioned in the History part earlier). The 2 styles are referring to Thailand's geographical and social dualism. The Southern style was practiced and developed by doctors, monks and practitioners of the ruling Royal family and class in Bangkok. The Northern style was carried and practiced by the local monks and folk healers treating the worker class in the northern part of the country. The subject of this book is the Northern style.

Thai massage is traditionally done on a floor mat where practitioner has the most leverage to use its own body. In Thailand, several different kinds of short tables are in use, most of them are shorter than knee height. One newer western variation of Thai massage is the Table Thai -that brings Thai massage exercises up onto the elevated massage table- is far from the traditional Thai massage. It is god for introducing the moves and exercises to the table bound public but looses all the benefits of the leverage that a practitioner have on a lower positioned workplace.

The anticipated massage techniques kneading, squeezing, strokes and oil usage are not relevant part of Thai Massage. It is partly because receivers are fully clothed during the massage session –originates from the fact that nudity was banned in the Thai temples (Wat) where massage has been practiced traditionally- and mostly because the practice is focused on the invisible energy system of the human body. Clearly the Indian yogis who explored and envisioned the Prana system and the Thais who gracefully selected the main energy lines out of it had unique intuitive skills to see and feel -and apply the rules of- the invisible currents of life-energy.

This energy body and the energy flow in it can be stimulated and influenced by pressing certain points along the channels of this invisible life-energy. Its specific techniques are palming and thumbing. Palm and thumb press used virtually all over the body with the exception of bony areas where straight pressure substituted with circular motion. Experienced advanced practitioners also use their feet, elbow, knee or their own bodyweight with ease. Thai massage also known about its stretches that vary from a local one joint stretch to the beautiful and impressive body wide stretches. Often the combination of pressure and stretch are used in the same exercise. These exercises are the subject of Part II.

The exotic atmosphere of Thai massage hinges on the delivery of the flow of the massage. The session is flowing when moves, exercises and their sequences are intuitively chosen, tailored for the receiver and transitions between exercises, and body positions are natural. Practitioner needs to be comfortable and confident in order to effectively perform these tasks. The best way to grow and maintain confidence is practicing. I mean practicing a lot! To maintain comfort during the lengthy massage sessions Thai massage employs positional and body mechanical standards for practitioners.

The basic principle of body mechanics is the usage of the maximum available body weight over the point of action with leverage by making the effort in every move and exercise to use bodyweight -in a sense of a lever as a simple machine where practitioner's body weight is balanced with the receiver's body and resistance- instead of using muscle strength. It saves energy, strength and avoids the often occurring hand, arm and back injury and overload. The optimal positions and moves for practitioners are as follows:

• Straight arms for palm or thumb press and for creating fulcrum for stretches
• Side to side rhythmic move of the upper body during palming and thumbing
• Positioning over and at the middle of receiver's body or body part
• Guiding moves from the center of the body, known as Hara
• Using the hips to initiate movements
• Borrowing elements from yoga, thai chi and other movement traditions

The last element of Thai massage is the place where the massage takes place. The studio or location needs to meet local rules and regulations and it of course determinates the clientel. A good floor mat, several differnet shaped pillows, good heating and cooling, natural sounds in the backround, small amount of aroma therapy in a form of insence or oil what will make the session a long lasting experience.

Thai massage has two different applications, the more available and popular energy balancing massage and the therapy. Originally Thai massage was utilized as a preventive and repetitive activity to maintain the even flow of the life-energy in the body. This evenness can be achieved by balancing the flow between stagnant areas of the body. It usually takes longer massage session and involves most of receiver's body. Receiving it feels good and has a general good sensation.

During energy balancing massage receiver should be relaxed and not "helping" the practitioner with movements and exercises. This kind of helping –which then improves into holding after helping has resolved- is influenced by stress, trauma and lack of trust. Therefore Thai massage is very good for people with conditions stemming from those issues.

The therapy application focuses on certain issues, conditions and locations or body parts. Its main goal to free the local blockage of stagnation of the life-energy flow. It usually takes shorter time but much more sensationful. The communication in such a treatment involves close feedback and rapport between practitioner and receiver. Traditional therapies know for knee pain, back ache, and neck pain. Often the two application can merge into one session and splitting the time, for example spending 1 ½ hour with energy balancing and ½ hour therapy focusing on a region or body part.

About this manual

The 2 hour, Full Body, Energy Balancing, Thai Yoga Massage.

This book balances the ancient techniques of Thai Yoga Massage and the mystical, somewhat foggy theories of the East with the scientific knowledge and insights of the West.

For the Western student, trying to learn a form consisting of 128 separate exercises without being taught underlying energetic, anatomic or kinesiological principles puts her mindset in the land of trust and intuition. For people growing up in a western society, like myself, it can be challenging and the learning curve seems to be steep. But by sticking with it and trusting yourself each exercise will reveal its benefits on the life-energy system and the physical structure of the human body. Be mindful that the challenges you will face while learning Thai Yoga Massage will also teach you many lessons about yourself.

Traditional Thai Theravada Buddhism, as the source and carrier of Thai Yoga Massage, is important on a religious and cultural level. But it is not necessary to be a Buddhist or hold to any specific faith tradition to practice or receive Thai Yoga Massage.

In my practice I relate to the yogic tradition and the teachings of Asokananda. He was the one who called his practice Thai Yoga Massage, a name that accurately describes this healing modality.

In our society, I am working to preserve and expancd roles for Thai Yoga Massage as a part of preventive medicine. I am also exploring a new way to reposition the wholistic nature of it by setting it within the framework of Structural Integration. Part III, Sen Line Anatomy, describes and analyzes the theoretical background of the Sen Lines of Thai Yoga Massage and its resemblance to the myofascial meridians.

TERMS USED IN THIS BOOK:

- The *Receiver* is the focus and is referred to as "her".
- *Inside* or *outside* in reference to a hand or leg refers to its closeness relative to the longitudinal midline of the receiver.
- *Half kneeling* or *lunge* with one knee on the floor is Warrior position.
- Two knees on the floor is kneeling.
- Diamond sitting is kneeling on your heels with toes curled under

- Posterior, anterior, medial, lateral, inferior, superior, distal and proximal are all anatomy terms and I use them whenever necessary.
- *Inside, outside* refers to medial and lateral side of receiver's leg. It will mainly describe the position of the Sen Energy Lines.
- *Point of resistance* is where the resistance of receiver kicks in. It is not the point where receiver starts to actively resist. That is the stretch reflex and it is recommended not to reach.
- The *dominant leg* is based on the traditional gender rule of Thai massage, where the Woman's dominant side is the Left and the Man's dominant side is the Right.
- *Outward* and *inward* will tell you which way the rotation should happen on the top of the body part
- The description of each exercise follows the Practitioner's Position (PP), Preparation (Prep), Exercise step by step (Exercise), Contraindications (Ci), Recommendations (Rec), Body mechanics (Bm), Effects (Eff), Hints to look for (Hints) and Sen Line (Sen Line) structure.
- (E) marks the Essential exercises

PART II
THE STRUCTURE OF THE 2 HOUR ENERGY BALANCING THAI YOGA MASSAGE
- Manual -

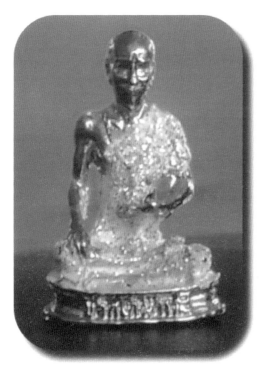

Meditative prayer

The traditional way of starting a massage is a short meditation standing, kneeling or sitting by the receiver to gather and express spirituality to yourself and to the greater power that you believe in. In Thai massage we pay respect to Jivaka Kumar Bhaccha the legendary founder of thaimassage and below you'll find the Om Namo Sivago mantra for it. The other mantra the Om Mani Padme Hum is a link to the yoga tradition through Tibet.

It's helpful to set your goals and intention for this session and keeping your mind clear and focused throughout this precious time of „Metta" loving kindness.

OM MANI PADME HUM
OM is the sound or vibration of the universe, a symbol for cosmic unity
MANI is jewel or diamond, symbolizing the shining light of love and compassion, as well as the power of the diamond, cutting through ignorance
PADME is a lotus flower symbolizing the ability to grow out of the mud and unfold into beauty, to grow out of the mud of ignorance and unfold into beauty of insight and enlightenment
HUM means to bring together, to unify
The lotus flower growing out of the mud is opening. A jewel in the center of the lotus flower gives out the shining light of compassion, which is connected with the sound of the cosmos, creating cosmic unity.

OM NAMO SHIVAGO SILASA AHANG
KARUNIKO
SAPASATANANG OSATHA TIPA-
MANTANG PAPASO
SURIYA-JANTANG
GOMALAPATO PAKA-SESI WANT AMI
BANTITO SUMETHASSO AROKHA
SUMANA-HOMI

PIYO-TEWA MANUSSANANG PIYO-PROMA
NAMUTTAMO
PIYO NAKHA SUPANANANG PININSIANG
NAMA-MIHANG
NAMO-PUTTAYA NAVON-NAVIEN
NASATIT-NASATIEN
EHI-MAMA NAVIEN-NAWE NAPATI-TANG-
VIEN
NAVIEN-MAHAKU EHI-MAMA PIYONG-
MAMA
NAMO-PUTTAYA
NA-A NA-WA ROKHA PAYATI VINA-SANTI.

Chapter 1
Foot massage and the
Sen Energy Lines of the leg

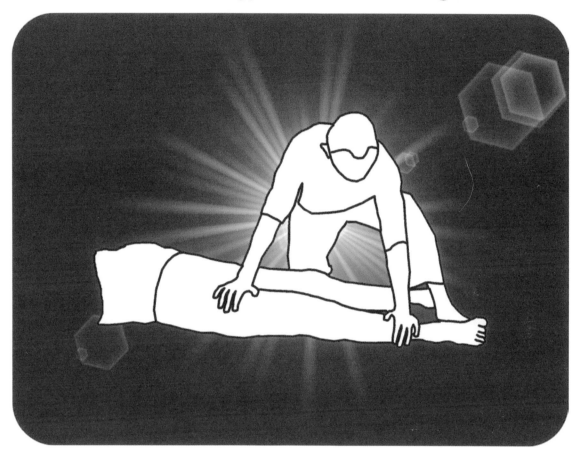

The foot massage and the work with the legs are traditionally the starting of the energy balancing session. The goal is to facilitate the energy flow from the limbs toward the main chakra system upward and ultimately to charge the crown chakra. When the flow of the energy is blocked or stagnant the living force and functions of the area decreasing and this condition become the source of other health issues.

This chapter introduces basic techniques and positions, simple stretches with the feet and application of the Sen Energy Lines and points along them.
The foot massage takes about 10 minutes in the session while working with the leg lines is about 20 minutes.

1. Foot massage

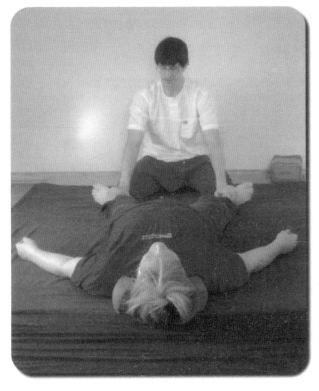

1.1 Palming the feet (E)

PP: Kneel by receiver's feet in diamond pose.

Exercise: Palm the medial feet with rocking motion from side to side.

Cover the whole medial part of both feet with alternated palming from the heel to the ball of the feet.

Rec: You are setting the speed and flow for the whole session now.

This first touch of the massage gives the initial information to receiver about you as a therapist.

Bm: Keep your arms straight and rock your upper body from side to side.

Eff: It loosens the feet and the ankles all the way up to the hips and abdomen.

Hints: This is a good time to look for restriction, flexibility, holding patterns throughout receiver's body.

Sen Line: *Sen Sumana*

1.2 Thumbing six points of the sole

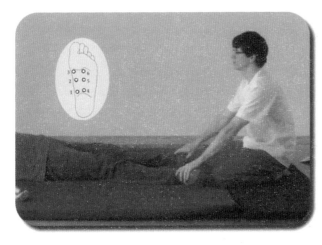

PP: Stay in the diamond position.

Prep: The six points of the sole cover acupressure zones related to intestines, the lungs, and most of the internal organs.

Exercise: Thumb press each of the 6 points simultaneously in the order of 1-2-3-2-1 then 4-5-6-5-4 on both feet to stimulate related organs and give receiver a sense of your firm touch.

Rec: Thaimassage doesn't recognize reflexology points but the stimulation of reflex zones easily fits into the practice of thaimassage.

Hints: You'll feel different textures in the underlaying tissues at different areas and points of the sole.

Sen Line: *Sen Kalathari*

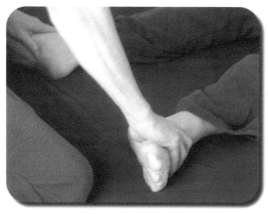

1.3 Thumbing medial arch

PP: Kneel by receiver's feet in diamond pose.
Exercise: Optionally thumb press medial arch of the feet simultaneously.
Eff: Thumbing the medial arch makes receiver feel good.
Sen Line: *Sen Sumana*

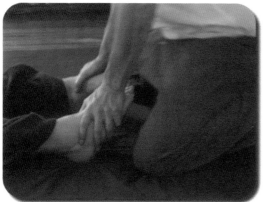

1.4 Palming in plantar flexion (E)

PP: Come to kneeling on both knees.
Prep: Turn receiver's feet inward so the toes will point upward.
Tuck the heels under by lifting and tilting the feet away from the body.
Exercise: Palm press the dorsum of both feet simultaneously from the ankle toward to the toes and back.

Rec: Usual pattern of palming is 1-2-3-2-1 at each segment of the body like the feet or lower, upper leg etc.
Bm: Again, use your upper body weight instead of your arm strength by leaning slightly forward and over the feet!
Sen Line: *Sen Kalathari*

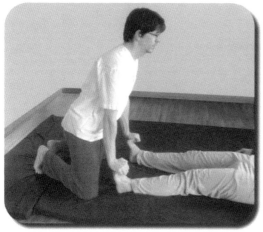

1.5 Dorsiflexion (E)

PP: Kneeling position
Prep: Place your palms on receiver's soles covering the ball of her feet.
Exercise: First push the ball of both feet simultaneously with your palms toward receiver's body to create a stretch throughout the posterior side of the leg. Then use your fingers to bend the toes toward the leg adding extra stretch while coming up and off of your heels to create a greater stretch with your body weight. Finish with the same push on the ball of the feet again.
Sen Line: *Sen Kalathari*

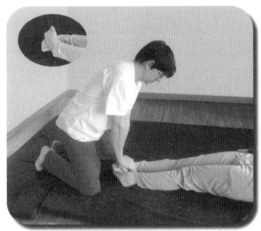

1.6 Pressing crossed feet (E)

PP: Kneeling

Prep: Test both feet individually by palm pressing them medially toward the floor.

Exercise: Choose the more flexible foot to repeat palm press and hold it down.

Grab receiver's other foot by its medial arch with your other hand and place it over the foot held down.

Now you have the two feet crossing on each other.

Place your palms on each other on the upper foot and press it down.

Eff: You're looking for a stretch over the dorsum of the feet but also creating an acupressure effect with the lower foot's cuneiform and metatarsal bones on the sole and reflex areas of the upper foot.

Sen Line: *Sen Kalathari*

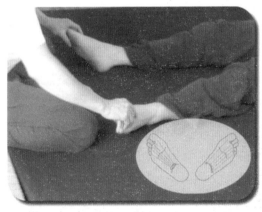

1.7 Thumbing from heel to toes

PP: In diamond sitting at receiver's feet.

Prep: You can choose thumbing the sole in fan direction or along paralell lines.

The fan starts from the middle point right front of the heel and spreads all the way to the toes like the plantar aponeuroses.

The paralell lines start from around the front of the heel and they cover most of the plantar fascia to the metatarsal-phalange joints.

Exercise: Start thumbing from the heel toward the big toe in a straight line.

Change thumb press to thumb circles when you approach the MP joint and phalanges.

Thumb circle the toe.

Finish with optional toe cracking or with pinching the tip of each toe.

Start from the heel again and repeat it in the directions of each toes.

Rec: Apply firm thumb pressure on the sole of the foot.

Eff: By covering the whole surface of the sole of the foot, the stimulation of reflex zones of the internal organs is well done.

Hints: Watch out for arthritis or swollen joints and apply appropriate gentle pressure.

Sen Line: *Sen Kalathari*

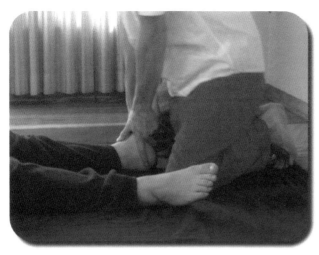

1.8 Thumb press ST41 with dorsiflexion

PP: From this point on it is more effective to work with one foot at the time.

Pick the one foot to start with, based on the gender rule (Women L, Men R) and kneel in line with it.

Prep: The point ST41 is between the foot and the leg front of the ankle joint in the indentation between the two deeper Extensor Hallucis Longus and Extensor Digitorum tendons.

Exercise: Hold the sole of the foot with your fingers and place your thumbs on the ST41.

Apply pressure with your thumbs on the point while dorsiflex the foot with your fingers.

Bm: The pressure over your thumbs should come through your arms and upper body by leaning slightly forward from your knees.

Sen Line: *Sen Kalathari*

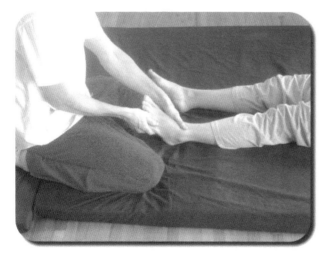

1.9 Thumb circles on top of the foot

PP: Kneeling

Exercise: Start with a double thumb press at the point ST41 front of the ankle.

Then circle your thumb following the tendons of the dorsum of the foot all the way to the tip of the toes.

Optionally repeat the pinch on the tip of each toe.

Eff: This great exercise warms up the foot.

Sen Line: *Sen Kalathari*

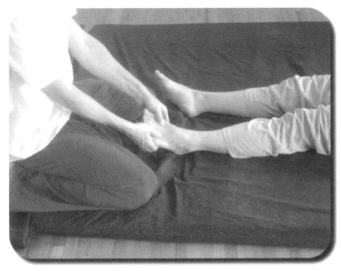

1.10 Thumb press between distal ends of metatarsals

PP: Kneeling
Prep: There are two reflex areas of the foot that we choose to work with.
Exercise: Press one thumb firmly between the metatarsals of the big toe and 2nd toe and your other thumb between the metatarsals of the little toe and the 4th toe.
Eff: These reflex areas represent the chest, upper back and the lungs. We are using them to stimulate energy flow of the foot and in the corresponding areas.
Hints: These points can be sensitive, but firm sinking pressure will be effective.
Sen Line: *Sen Kalathari*

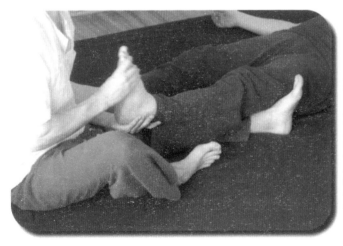

1.11 Ankle rotation both directions (E)

PP: Sittting with inside leg straight, outside leg bent.
Prep: Cup receiver's heel with your inside hand and place your other thumb on the solar plexus just below the ball of the foot.
Hold the foot between your thumb and fingers.
Exercise: Rotate the foot first outward 3 times around then repeat the rotation 3 times to the opposite direction.
Lead the rotation with your upper body through firm thumb pressure on the solar plexus.
Rec: Slow down and reduce rotation when you are experiencing clicks, pops or grinding sound or sensation in the ankle.
Bm: Use your upper body to lead the rotation.
Sen Line: *Multiple*

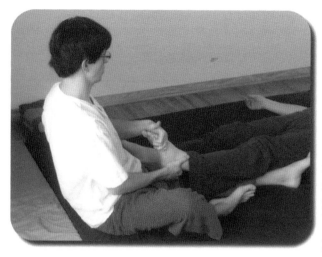

1.12 Twisting the foot laterally and medially with leaning back(E)

PP: Sittting with inside leg straight, outside leg bent.

Prep: Slide your outside hand medially onto the medial arch of the foot while holding the heel with your inside cup hand.

Exercise: Grab the foot at the medial arch and lean back with your upper body to twist the foot laterally.

Repeat twist with moving your hand in different position on the medial arch between the heel and the ball of the foot.

Exchange hand positions and repeat the exercise this time grabbing the lateral arch of the foot and twist it medially.

Eff: By twisting the foot you're stretching the leg and hip and the side of the receiver's upper body.

Hints: Look for restrictions as your pull and twist travels through receiver's body.

Sen Line: *Sen Sumana (medial arch), Sen Ittha-Pingkhala (lateral arch)*

Repeat 1.11 on the same foot!

Repeat 1.8-1.12 on the other foot!

1.13 Cracking toes

Hint: Cracking toes is highly optional, consult with receiver before attempting it.

2. The Sen Energy Lines of the legs

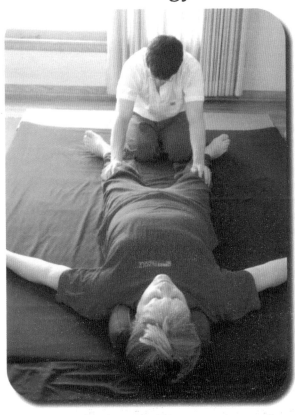

2.1 Palming medial legs up and down with palm circles on knees

PP: Kneeling by the receiver's feet.

Prep: This transition move is great to connect the looser feet and ankles to the rest of the legs and to the hips energetically by introducing your touch to these areas.

Kneeling by the feet you have the full length of the legs in reach.

You are able to cover the medial side of the feet and the lower leg, the anterior side of the knee with the patella and the anterior-medial side of the thighs.

Exercise: Starting with palming the medial feet by rocking your upper body from side to side as you done it before during the foot massage.

Then move on the medial side of the heel and continue palming upward on the medial surface of the lower leg.

Substitute palm press on the knees with 3-5 palm circles at the knees simultaneously and outward.

Approaching the thighs you need to lift up from sitting on your heels to reach them.

Then keep moving onto the thighs just below the groin.

From here turn back and continue the palming all the way down to the feet and toes with palm circles on the knees again.

Rec: The substitution of palming follows one of the rules of thaimassage: "do not press on bone"

Bm: Utilize your upper body weight throughout the palming by shifting your position from sitting to kneeling.

Eff: This is one of the simplest and most calming beginner transition move.

Hints: Sense the holding pattern and tightness of the Rectus Femoris and underlying tissues.

Sen Line: *Sen Kalathari,*
Sen Sahatsarangsi-Thawari

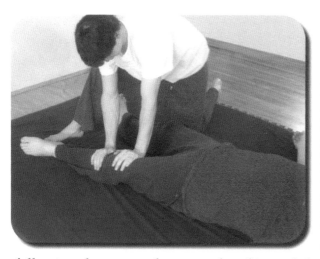

2.2 Palming medial leg (E)

PP: Follow the gender rule and approach the inside of the dominant leg in half kneeling over the closer leg from receiver's opposite side.

Prep: The 3 lines of the medial leg run longitudinal, emerging from the foot and crossing the ankle and the knee to connect up to the hip.

The *1st* inside line runs from below the ankle bone parallel to the tibia following the groove between the tibia and the exposed edge of the Soleus up to the medial condyle of the tibia. It stretches over the medial edge of the knee joint to the corner of the patella and up following the groove between Rectus Femoris and Vastus Medialis muscle. The line then continues from the groin upward.

The *2nd* line is also emerging from the foot just posterior to or "below" the ankle bone from the soft spot that "covered" by the so called felxor retinaculum. It runs parallel to the *1st* line following the tendon of the Gastrocnemius to the medial knee.

It passes the knee to the indentation between the vastus medialis and the adductor group to go on the inner thigh following the anterior septum between Vastus Medialis and Adductor muscles.

This line also continues from the groin up.

The *3rd* line is a continuation from the middle line of the heel all the way up to behind the knee following the achilles tendon.

It pases the back of the knee and follows the mid line of the back of the thigh.

A branch line splits out and became the *3rd* inside line of the inner thigh following the Gracilis muscles to join the midline of the torso by the perineum.

Exercise: Start palming the full length of the inner leg with one hand from the ankle and the other hand from the groin.

Palm to the knee with both hands, then palm back to the starting points.

Then palm back to the knee again and palm down all the way to the ankle with both hands.

Palm gentle but firmly and monitor receiver's feedback for pressure.

Rec: Back in time Thai massage was a major part of people's life due to agricultural lifestyle. Working with the leg was a crucial part of practice.

Bm: Keep your knee outside of your arms to allow yourself using your upper body and keep your own energy flowing.

Open and use your hips to tansfer your bodyweight from one hand to the other.

Eff: This is a simple and relaxing palming sequence for the sensitive inner thigh. It prepares the leg for the thumbing.

Sen Line: *Multiple*

2.3 Thumbing medial leg (3 lines) (E)

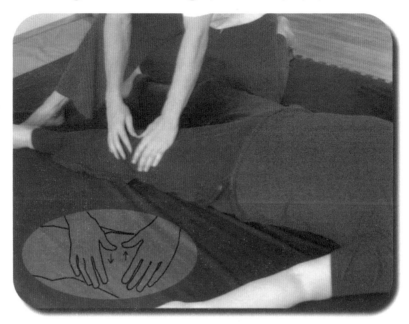

PP: In half kneeling position place both of your hands at receiver's ankle.

Prep: The simple thumbing technique is the thumb-chasing-thumb style when one thumb moving ahead following the energy line and the other thumb "chases" it.

Touching the 2 thumbs together during thumbing is important for connecting the flow of energy.

Exercise: Thumb the *1st* inside line from the ankle to below the knee and back to the ankle.

Switch to the *2nd* line and thumb the same way up to below the knee and back to the ankle.

And yes, switch to the *3rd* line and thumb up to below the back of the knee and back to the ankle.

Change your position up closer to receiver's torso with palming from ankle to above the knee.

Thumb the thigh between the knee and the hip in similar order, *1st*, *2nd* and *3rd* inside Energy lines as you did with the lower leg.

Ci: Serious varicose veins are contraindicated and thumbing could leave bruise like dark marks on the leg with cellulite.

Bm: Rock your upper body gently from your stretching hip and legs to use it as leverage over your thumbs.

Eff: Thumbing greatly induces energy flow throughout the body. It specifically brings the energy up from the limbs toward the chakra system ultimately to energize the crown chakra.

Sen Line: *Multiple*

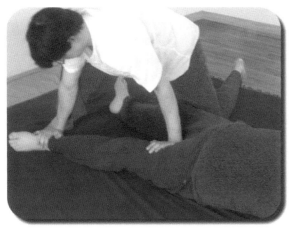

2.4 Stretch and press medial leg (3 lines) (E)

PP: Sittting with inside leg straight, outside leg bent.

Prep: Cup receiver's heel with your inside hand and place your other thumb on the solar plexus just below the ball of the foot.

Hold the foot between your thumb and fingers.

Exercise: Rotate the foot first outward 3 times around then repeat the rotation 3 times to the opposite direction. Lead the rotation with your upper body through firm thumb pressure on the solar plexus.

Rec: Slow down and reduce rotation when you are experiencing clicks, pops or grinding sound or sensation in the ankle.

Bm: Use your upper body to lead the rotation.

Sen Line: *Multiple*

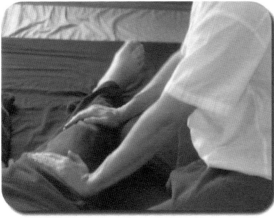

2.5 Palming lateral leg(E)

PP: Move back by sitting on your heels outside of receiver's other leg.

Prep: Front of you is the lateral side of receiver's other leg.

Position yourself to the middle in level with the knee, to able to reach both end of the leg.

In prone position the *1st* and *2nd* outside lines are easily accessible the *3rd* line rather out of reach.

Exercise: Palm the outside surface of the leg the same way as you palmed the inside previously.

Start with your hands at the ankle and at the proximal end of the thigh and palm with rocking motion from side to side toward the knee and palm back to the starting positions.

Then back to the knee again just to palm away to the ankle for transitioning and connecting to the upcoming thumbing.

Rec: During palming keep reciver's leg fixed as much as you can to avoid rolling it in and out.

Bm: Again, use your upper body weight to apply pressure and keep your arms straight.

Hints: Look for the resistance of the leg and holding pattern, also sense the tightness of the tissues.

Sen Line: *Multiple*

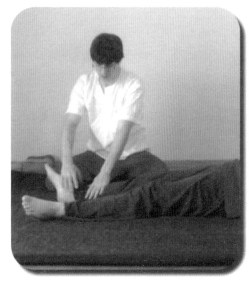

2.6 Thumbing lateral leg (2 lines) (E)

PP: Move your position a bit toward the foot to face the lower leg.

Prep: The *1st* line connecting the energy form and to the foot through the point ST41.

It leads up to the knee between the anterior edge of the tibia and the Tibialis Anterior muscle.

The *2nd* line passes just above the ankle bone and runs parallel to the *1st* line in the septum of the lateral compartment.

Above the knee the *1st* line continues from the corner of the patella and runs in the groove between the rectus femoris and vastus lateralis muscle into the hip.

The *2nd* line follows the Vastus Lateralis muscle front of the IT band from side of the knee to the hip.

Exercise: Thumb the *1st* outside line of the lower leg from the ankle to the knee and back then switch to the *2nd* line and repeat thumbing in the same pattern.

Then palm your way up to the knee and thumb the 2 energy lines of the thigh in similar pattern from knee to hip and back.

Bm: Use the side to side rocking movement while keep your elbows straight.

Sen Line: *Multiple*

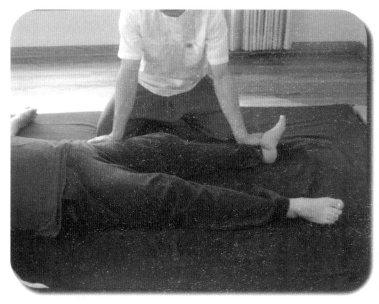

2.7 Stretch and press lateral leg (2 lines) (E)

PP: Move back to the middle of the leg in level with the knee to be able to reach both ends of the leg again.

Exercise: Place your palms on the ankle and on the proximal end of the thigh and press your arms away from the knee. First cover the *1st* outside line then the *2nd* outside line.

Sen Line: *Multiple*

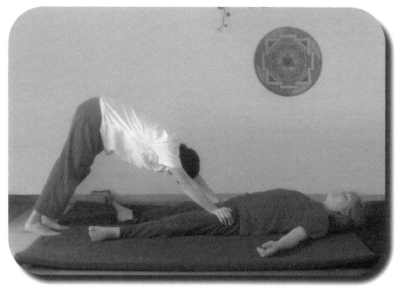

2.8 Blood stop

PP: Kneel by receiver's feet in the diamond position.

Prep: Palm up on the legs as you did before in *Exercise 2.1* but stop at the groin.

Very gentle place your palms on the groin and palpate the pulse of the two iliac arteries. It takes about 5-10 seconds to feel the pulse.

Exercise: When you clearly palpate the pulse on both sides, move your hands down to the thigh about an inch and cover the femoral artery with your palm.

Now you are in kneeling position which is powerful enough for most of receivers.

If you want to increase the blood stop you can move into the downward dog while keep holding the pulse.

Then you can move to the plank pose to apply even greater pressure.

Ci: Any kind of non-regular heart or circulatory condition prohibits the blood stop. Low or high blood pressure, heart disease or pacemaker etc.

Rec: Due to contraindications blood stop is not an essential exercise as it was back in time, since the overall cardiac health of receivers declined.

Bm: The downward dog and the plank require great sense of balance, flexibility and strength. Perform these only if you have these skills.

Normally the kneeling pose is plenty for both receivers and givers.

Eff: The blood stop increases the heart rate and the pressure in the vascular system. The traditional theory is to clean the "pipes " the veins and arteries by increasing the pressure then consequently letting the blocked blood retake them. This procedure known as the elimination of toxins from the blood flow.

Sen Line: *Sen Kalathari*

Chapter 2
Single leg exercises

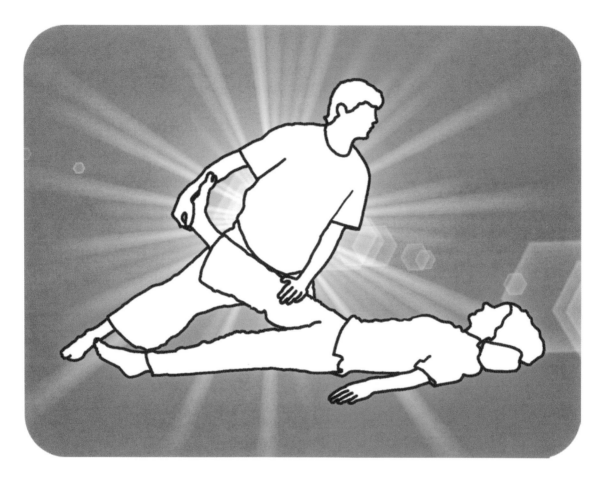

The single leg exercises are the most active and moving part of the session. Most of the exercises are great for stiff receivers and even yoga people will find them sensationful.
This chapter contains more than 25 individual exercises that give you plenty of options to work with different body types and sizes of receivers.
Working with one leg at the time gives therapist the opportunity to compare receiver's left and right sides which can yield the strategy for the rest of the session.
In the session you need to be selective and mindful choosing single leg exercises based on receiver's condition and the time you want to spend. This part of the sessiontakes at least 20 minutes.

3. Single leg exercises

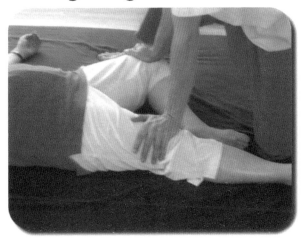

3.1 Palming both thighs in Tree pose

PP: From kneeling position to half kneeling

Prep: Pick up receiver's foot and place it by the other knee to open the bent leg to the side into the Tree yoga pose.

Move closer up to the bent knee and pick up your outside knee to get into a half kneeling lunge position.

Place your hands just above the knees on the thighs.

Exercise: Palm up and down both thighs alternated.

Rec: Be gentle with this palming. The intention is to introduce and relax receiver into this pose.

Eff: Opens hip and relaxes inner thigh hip region.

Hints: Receivers with stiffer hip and/or inner thigh will hold their knee.

Sen Line: *Multiple*

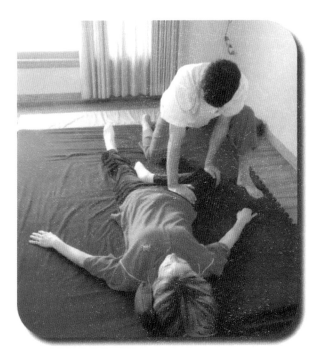

3.2 Palming bent medial leg in Tree pose (E)

PP: Staying in the lunge stance.

Prep: Move in line with the bent leg.

Place your outside cup hand on the knee of the bent leg for support.

Exercise: Start from the groin palm the inside thigh down to the knee and up to the groin.

Repeat palming up and down couple of times then optionally extend the palming to the lower leg.

Rec: If bent leg doesn't touch the floor use pillows for support.

The inner thigh can be sensitive so monitor receiver's feedback for your pressure.

Sen Line: *Sen Kalathari*

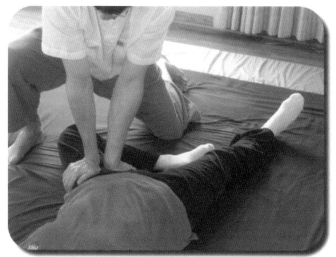

3.3 Butterfly palming bent medial thigh

PP: In lunging by receiver's bent leg turn your stance and attention to the inner thigh of the bent leg.

Prep: Put your hands together to form a "butterfly".

Leave space between your hands.

Exercise: Palm the inner thigh of the bent leg with both hands from the groin to the knee and back.

Sen Line: *Multiple*

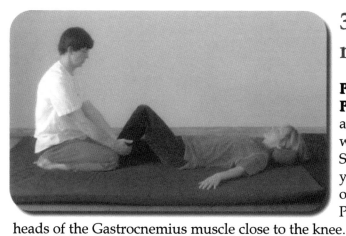

3.4 Separate calf muscles

PP: Kneel by receiver's feet.

Prep: Pull receiver's bent knee up away from the floor into vertical with her foot on the floor.

Stabilize receiver's foot between your thighs or by placing your foot on top of receiver's foot.

Place your fingers between the two heads of the Gastrocnemius muscle close to the knee.

Exercise: Pull your fingers toward yourself by leaning backward while support receiver's foot and lower leg so receiver's heel stays on the floor.

Repeat this move down and up on the lower leg.

Rec: The lower leg can be sensitive as tremendous tension can be held here. The calf muscles also can be ropy, stringy or stiff.

Bm: Lean back.

Sen Line: *Sen Sumana*

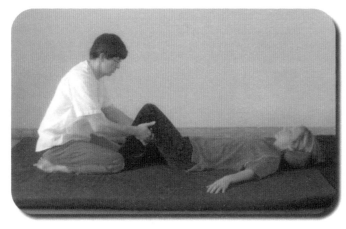

3.5 Push away calf muscles from bones

PP: Kneeling with holding receiver's foot between your knees.

Prep: Interlace your fingers behind receiver's lower leg.

Cover the posterior compartment of the lower leg with your plams.

Exercise: Squeez calf muscles with your palms and push away from Tibia and Fibula.

Rec: This exercise has a great effect when you do it with firm but not strong pressure.

Eff: Loosens the calf and releases the different layers of tissues.

Sen Line: *Sen Kalathari*

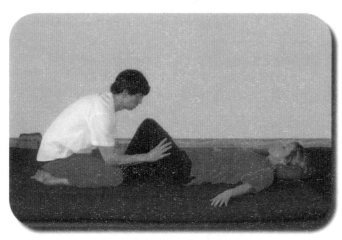

3.6 Thumbing hamstrings

PP: Kneeling with holding receiver's foot between your knees.

Prep: Lean a bit forward to brace receiver's thigh from underneath and place your thumbs on the back sid eof the thigh.

Your thumbs should reach all the way down to the midline of the thigh.

Exercise: Start thumbing from behind the knee and thumb as far as you can reach then thumb and back to the knee.

Rec: Be careful with the double thumb pressure as it can be quite strong. Apply pressure gradually.

Sen Line: *Sen Sumana*

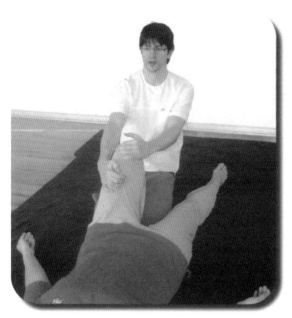

3.7 Twist bent leg's thigh with leaning back

PP: Kneeling with holding receiver's foot between your knees.

Prep: Push receiver's foot of her bent knee closer to her body to create better leverage.
Place your inside hand on receiver's knee.
Place the fingers of your outside hand by the medial superior corner of the patella.

Exercise: Hook your fingers into receiver's thigh then lean back and twist your hand in the same time.
Your outside hand working with the 1st inside Energy Line of the thigh.
Repeat this move down the thigh and back to the knee again.

Then change your hands, put your outside hand on the knee and your inside hand on the lateral superior corner of the patella.

Repeat leaning back and twisting your hand on receiver's thigh with your inside hand now working with the *1st* outside Energy Line of the thigh.

Bm: The twist should come from your upper body leaning back and not from your arm.

Sen Line: *Sen Sahatsarangsi-Thawari*

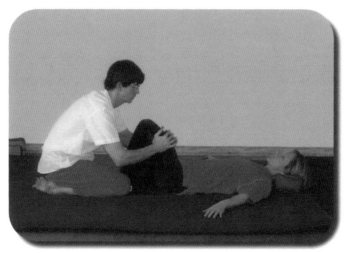

3.8 Push away Quadriceps muscles from Femur

PP: Kneeling with holding receiver's foot between your knees.

Prep: Interlace your fingers over receiver's thigh.

Exercise: Squeez receiver's thigh with your palms, following the 1-2-3-2-1 pattern down and up on the thigh.

Sen Line: *Sen Kalathari*

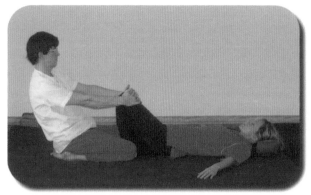

3.9 Stretch bent leg away with leaning back

PP: Kneeling with holding receiver's foot between your knees.

Prep: Place your hands on receiver's bent knee and interlace your fingers.

Exercise: Lean back and pull receiver's knee toward yourself all the way to the point of resistance.

You can hold the stretch for a while and then release back to the starting position.

Repeat with changing your hand position closer to the groin then back to the knee with each pull.

Rec: This exercise is hard to perform on receiver with stiff hips as the tightness will hold the hip back from extension.

Bm: Lean back.

Eff: Opens the front of the hip. Loosens hip flexors.

Sen Line: *Sen Sahatsarangsi-Thawari*

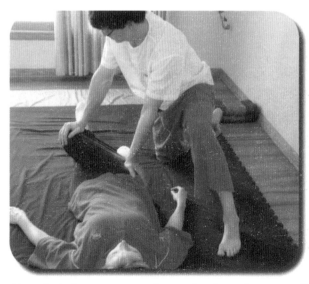

3.10 Cross stretch(E)

PP: Half kneel in the side of receiver's body.

Prep: Push receiver's bent leg over her straight leg all the way to the point of resistance.

Hold the knee of the bent leg in the cross stretch with one hand and place your other hand on the side of receiver's hip.

Exercise: Palm your way toward the knee and back with one hand while keep the leg stable in the stretch with your other hand.

Rec: It is important to keep the bent leg stretched and fixed during palming so it won't wobble and distract the flow.

Bm: Balance yourself with receiver's bent leg.

Eff: Streches the IT band, loosens the hip.

Sen Line: *Sen Kalathari*

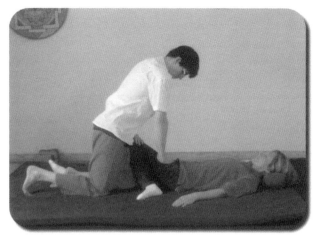

3.11 Thigh stretch with palming

PP: Kneeling by receiver's straight leg.
Prep: Push receiver's bent knee toward her chest with your inside hand.
Push the foot hanging in the air to the side with your outside hand's dorsal surface while letting the knee coming to your thighs in a circular move.
In the same time rise up and secure receiver's knee in the angle that appropriate for receiver's flexibility.
Exercise: Secure receiver's knee with your thigh and hand.
Palm the upper surface of receiver's thigh following the 1-2-3-2-1 pattern.
Release the leg the by pushing the knee toward the chest in a circular motion.
Rec: It is a complex exercise.
Always move the knee in circular motion.
Finding the proper angle for receiver's bent leg is the key.
Sen Line: *Sen Sahatsarangsi-Thawari*

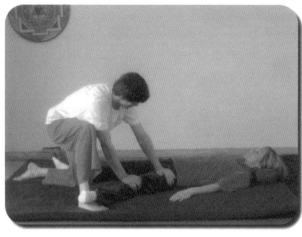

3.12 Bowling(E)

PP: Half kneeling by receiver's feet.
Prep: Straight receiver's leg out and hold it underneath the ankle with your outside hand.
Exercise: Step outside into the lunge stance and push receiver's leg into abduction.
When you are balanced in the lunge stance push back and forth receiver's leg to full abduction all the way to the point of resistance in 2-3 swings.
After reaching the point of resistance pull receiver's leg back to a comfortable position and place it on the dorsum of your lunging foot.
Place your outside hand on receiver's knee for support.
Palm receiver's inner thigh with your inside hand following the 1-2-3-2-1 pattern from knee to groin.
Rec: It is a fun and moving exercise. Play with it.
Eff: Opens hip, stretches inside of the leg, creates flow.
Sen Line: *Sen Kalathari*

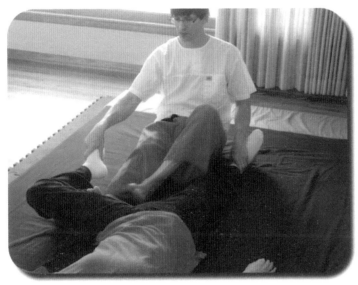

3.13 Single grape press(E)

PP: Sitting by receiver's feet.

Prep: Open receiver's knee to the side so her leg is in 90 degrees angle with her waist.

Hold on the foot of the bent leg with your outside hand and sit between receiver's bent and straight legs.

Place your feet on receiver's bent inner thigh close to the knee.

Hold receiver's straight leg with your other hand at the ankle.

Adjust your sitting to be able to reach the waist line with your straight leg.

Exercise: Push your outside foot forward to stretch receiver's bent leg.

Then release bent leg back with holding against it with your inside foot.

Adjust your outside foot on receiver's thigh closer to the hip and repeat the push to stretch the bent leg again.

Do this exercise as many time as you need with frequently changing your foot position on receiver's thigh.

Rec: Hold the foot of the bent leg in the air to allow it go back and forth freely.

Do this exercise sequence in every session.

This is one of receivers' favorite stretch. After receiving it you'll know why.

Your outside hand is strictly holding receiver's bent leg.

Do not pull or control the movement with your arm strength.

Bm: The rhythm of this exercise is crucial.

You need to use your upper body, legs and arms coordinated.

Eff: This exercise is the first in the sequence when receiver exposed to the moving nature of Thai massage.

Working with the often stiff posterior thigh the effect is incredible.

Sen Line: *Sen Sumana*

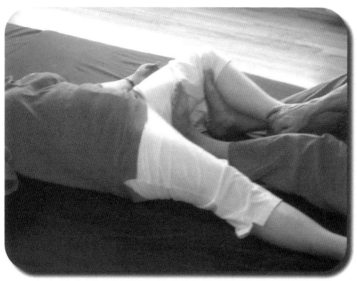

3.14 Twisted wine (leg locked for support) (E)

PP: Sitting by receiver's feet.

Prep: Place receiver's bent leg back to the 90 degrees angle and place your outside foot behind the bent knee to support it.

Move receiver's foot inward across over your lower leg into a lock.

Cup hand receiver's heel under your knee to hold this lock together.

Place your inside foot on receiver's inner thigh beside your other foot.

Exercise: Follow the 1-2-3-2-1 pattern with your inside foot pressing receiver's inner thigh while you holding resistance with the lock against it.

Bm: Pay attention to your own back and keep yourself straight up.

Eff: Releases hamstrings.

Sen Line: *Sen Sumana*

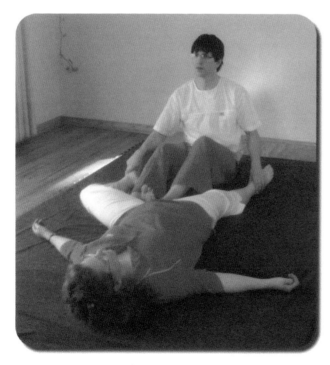

3.15 Double grape press(E)

PP: Sitting by receiver's feet.

Prep: Place both of your feet on receiver's bent inner thigh close to the knee and hold her foot fixed with your outside hand.

Place your other hand on receiver's other foot.

Exercise: Walk your feet back and forth on receiver's inner thigh between the knee and the hip applying gentle pressure.

Rec: It should be relaxing and firm feeling for receiver and you can be playful with this exercise.

Sen Line: *Sen Sumana*

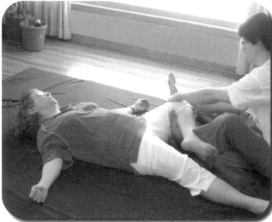

3.16 Twist and pull the thigh of the bent leg with foot support

PP: Sitting by receiver's feet.

Prep: Place your inside foot behind receiver's bent knee for support while relaxing your outside leg away from receiver.

Pull receiver's bent lower leg across your supporting leg into a lock.

Keep receiver's bent leg in a 90 degrees angle and place your outside hand on her knee and your inside hand just above the knee reaching over to the lateral side of her thigh.

Exercise: Hook your 4 fingers into receiver's lateral thigh and apply firm pull by leaning backward.

Follow the lateral side of her thigh up to the hip pulling and releasing then return to the starting position with the same motion.

Bm: Sometime it is difficult to get into this position so remember to open your bent leg to allow yourself to get closer.

Sen Line: *Sen Sahatsarangsi-Thawari*

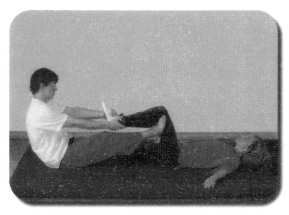

3.17 Knee stretch with hamstring press

PP: Sitting by receiver's feet.

Prep: Close receiver's bent knee up over the hip and grab receiver's heel and foot with both hands.

Place your inside leg over receiver's straight leg and position your other foot below receiver's bent knee on the back of her thigh.

Exercise: Apply firm press with your foot on her thigh.

When you push with your foot you need to resist and pull receiver's foot with your hands.

Follow the 1-2-1 pattern with slow motion and take your time for each press to allow this stretch effect deeper.

Ci: Knee replacement and history of serious knee injury is contraindicated.

Rec: Keep receiver's bent leg in the 90 degrees angle during the exercises.

Bm: Lean back and extend your leg in the same time to create the motion and the stretch.

Sen Line: *Sen Sumana*

3.18 1-2-3 hip lift

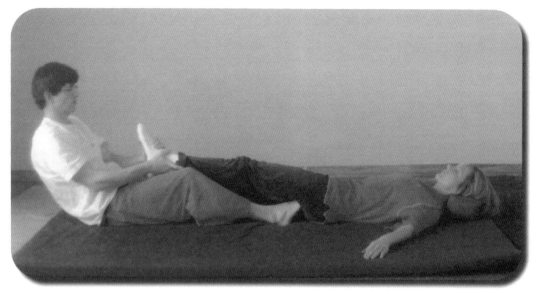

PP: Sitting by receiver's feet.

Prep: Set receiver's bent knee over her hip again and plant your foot between the floor and receiver's bent leg so your foot resting on the back of her thigh like on a pedal.

Hold receiver's foot with both hands.

Throw your other leg over receiver's straight leg.

During this exercise keep your foot under receiver's bent leg.

Exercise: Push receiver's bent leg forward like a knee to chest exercise and pin the ball of your foot on her thigh.

Pull the whole leg toward yourself by leaning back.

Without holding return to the starting position.

Then push receiver's bent leg further ahead so your toes will slide lower on her thigh.

Pin the ball of your foot your foot again on her thigh and lean back.

Bend receiver's leg again to push it all the way as far as you can this time to allow your toes sliding down all the way to the Ischial Tuberosity.

Gently pull receiver's leg into extension by leaning back and eventually find yourself in lying on the floor stretching out horizontally.

Ci: Hip replacement.

Rec: You got to be careful with this exercise especially with stiff people who will not able to go to the full extension due to their stiff hip and hipflexors.

Take them only to the point of resistance and let them relax in that position.

Eff: This is a great exercise to stretch the hip and the quads. The stretch effect the hip flexors and the hamstrings while giving a brake to the lower back and most importantly adjust the relative position of the two sides of the hip.

Hints: Sens release in the hip with each extentions.

Sen Line: *Sen Sumana*

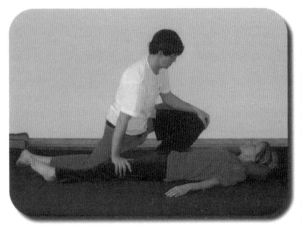

3.19 Knee to chest hand on straight leg's thigh(E)

PP: Half kneeling in line with receiver.

Prep: Get into half kneel facing toward receiver with your front foot beside receiver's hip.

Bend her knee to place her foot into the top of your groin.

Place your outside hand on receiver's bent knee and your inside hand on her straight leg on the thigh.

Exercise: Extend your lunge by moving your hip and upper body forward to push receiver's bent leg forward and her knee toward her chest.

Palm receiver's other thigh to balance and increase the stretch in the hip and legs.

Follow the 1-2-3-2-1 pattern to move your hand on receiver's thigh while repeating the knee to chest push.

Rec: It is a challenge that reveals who is more flexible as you are reflexions of each other in the position.

Sen Line: *Multiple*

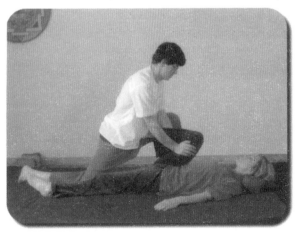

3.20 Knee to chest hands on posterior thigh

PP: Half kneeling.

Prep: Hold receiver's foot with your groin.

Place your butterfly hands on posterior side of receiver's thigh.

This exercise is a variation of the single leg version of the Knee to chest exercise(3.19).

Exercise: Repeat the knee to chest exercise with the enforcement of your palming hands on receiver's thigh with a 1-2-1 pattern.

Rec: Very effective exercise for stiff or heavy receivers to stretch and mobilize the hamstrings and the lower back.

Sen Line: *Sen Sumana*

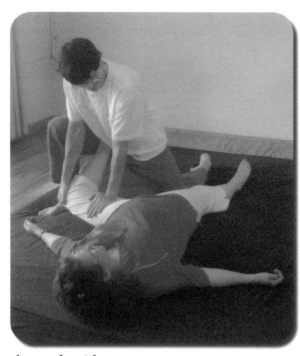

3.21 Knee to the side with palming the medial bent thigh

PP: Half kneeling.
Prep: This exercise is the 2nd variation for the Knee to chest exercise.
Open receiver's bent leg to the side.
Place your outside hand on receiver's knee and your inside hand on the inner thigh of her bent leg.
Exercise: Palm receiver's inner thigh while stretch her bent leg toward the floor and not so much forward.
Follow the 1-2-3-2-1 pattern with the palming and support the bent leg's foot with your groin.
Rec: Pay attention when open the bent leg to the side.
Strong holding patterns can be exposed.
Eff: This is a great exercise to stretch the often tight inner thigh and hip.
Sen Line: *Sen Sumana*

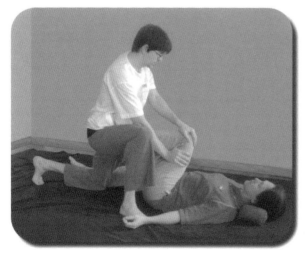

3.22 Knee to opposite shoulder with palming 3rd outside line

PP: Half kneeling.
Prep: Put your inside hand on receiver's knee and your outside hand on the outside of her bent leg's thigh.
Hold receiver's foot with your groin.
Exercise: Push receiver's leg forward and across toward her opposite shoulder while palm on her bent leg's hamstrings following the 1-2-3-2-1 pattern.
Hints: This exercise has known to create deep stretch in the hip jont. Monitor receiver's feedback and skip exercise if pain occur.
Sen Line: *Sen Ittha-Pingkhala*

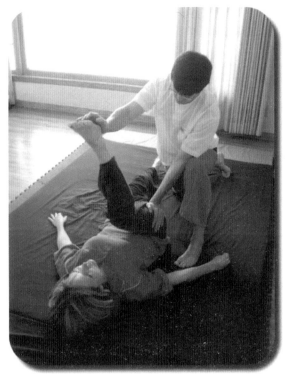

3.23 Rocking horse original

PP: Half kneeling.

Prep: Bend receiver's leg by holding at the heel with your inside hand's cupping and your outside hand at the back of her thigh.

Exercise: Push the heel forward by extending your arm with lunging forward from your hip.

Palm with your other hand receiver's posterior thigh simultaneously with the forward move then release and get back to the starting position.

Follow the 1-2-3-2-1 pattern palming with lunging forward.

Rec: The most stretch should occur between your hands in receiver's leg by pinning the thigh and extending the lower leg away.

Bm: The main feature of this exercise is the rhythm rather than the force. If you do it right receiver's straight leg will come up from the floor.

Sen Line: *Sen Ittha-Pingkhala*

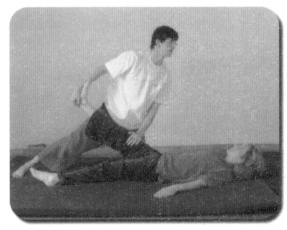

3.24 Posterior leg stretch with upper body twist

PP: Half kneeling.

Prep: Hold receiver's leg with cup hand at the heel with your inside hand so your forearm will hold the plantar surface of the foot.

Turn your kneeling toward receiver's legs by kneel with your outside leg by her hip and picking up your inside leg and straight it out.

Rest your outside hand on receiver's thigh just above the knee.

Exercise: Slightly lift receiver's leg and turn with your upper body toward receiver.

Eff: Your upper body turn creates the stretching over the plantar surface of receiver's foot and all the way up on the posterior side of the leg.

Sen Line: *Sen Sumana*

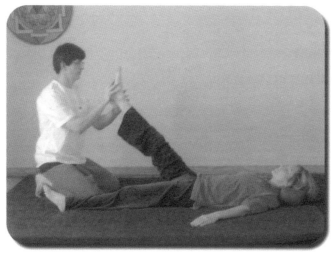

3.25.1 One leg lift(E)

PP: Kneel by receiver's feet.
Prep: Pick up receiver's leg with both hands.
Exercise: Push straight leg forward and up while keeping it straight then release it back down to the floor.
Rec: This variation is designed for stiff or elderly receivers whose range of motion is limited.
If you can lift receiver's leg up easially with no resistance use a different variation of this exercise as described later.
Hints: Do not push over the vertical angle even if receiver is that flexible.
Sen Line: *Sen Sumana*

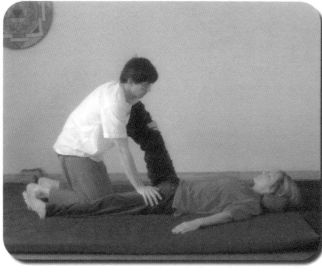

3.25.2 One leg lift on shoulder with hand support on straight leg

PP: Come up to half kneeling and place receiver's elevated leg on your outside shoulder.
Prep: The posterior side of receiver's heel should fit just right on top of your shoulder.
Hug receiver's thigh above or below the knee with your outside hand and place your inside hand on receiver's straight leg to support and stablize yourself.
Exercise: Slowly move your body forward to push reciever's leg up and forward.
When you reach the point of resistance or start feeling receiver shaking release and move back to the starting position.
Rec: Do one full stretch and move on. Do not repeat this exercise many times.
Sen Line: *Sen Sumana*

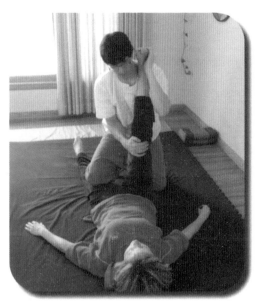

3.25.3 One leg lift on shoulder with thigh support on straight leg

PP: Kneeling in line of receiver's thighs.
Prep: Place your outside hand on the plantar surface of receiver's foot on your shoulder and hug the knee with your inside hand.
Balance yourself and place your knee on receiver's straight thigh for deeper stretch .
Exercise: Slowly come up and lean forward to stretch the back of the leg and the lower back.
When you reach the point of resistance or start feeling receiver shaking release and move back to the starting position.
Rec: Never stretch receiver's leg over the vertical angle.
Sen Line: *Sen Sumana*

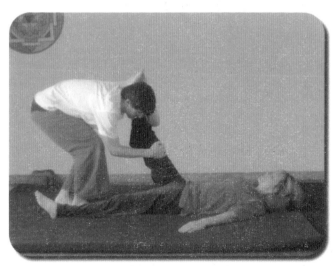

3.25.4 One leg lift on shoulder in standing

PP: Standing by receiver's feet.
Prep: Pick up receiver's foot and place it on your outside shoulder.
To be able to do this you probably need to bend forward and bend your knees.
Your upper body will be more or less horizontal.
Secure receiver's foot on your shoulder with your outside hand and brace the knee with your inside hand.
Exercise: Slowly shift your position forward to stretch the leg on your shoulder and come back to the starting position.
Rec: Do not go and stretch receiver's leg over the vertical angle with this exercise. You can easily lose your balance by going too far ahead with a very flexible receiver.
Bm: Pay attention to your lower back. Keep your back straight as much as you can. If you feel discomfort in your back doing this exercise just skip it.
Hints: Look for balance.
Sen Line: *Sen Sumana*

3.25.5 One leg lift on shoulder in standing balancing with straight leg

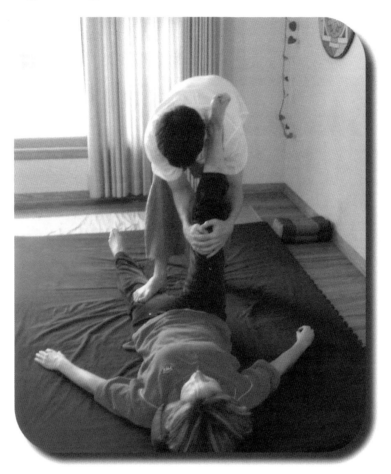

PP: Standing by receiver's feet.

Prep: Pick up receiver's foot and place it on your outside shoulder.

To be able to do this you probably need to bent forward and bend your knees.

Your upper body will be more or less horizontal.

Find your balance and rest your inside foot on receiver's other thigh.

It is important not to step on receiver's thigh but rather balancing yourself with it.

Secure receiver's foot on your shoulder by bracing the knee with your hands.

Exercise: Shift your body forward adding extra stretch with your foot on receiver's other thigh then release by shifting back to the starting position.

Rec: Only do this stretch once.

Bm: This exercise requires great balance and sensitivity. You can prepare your skills and senses by practicing the easier variations of One leg lift.

Sen Line: *Sen Sumana*

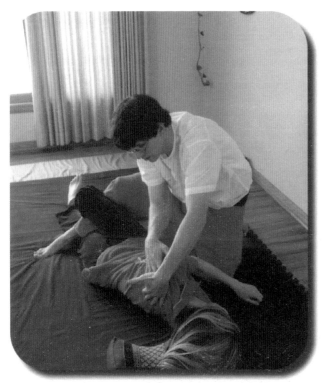

3.26 Spinal twist with pivot knee leverage(E)

PP: Half kneel beside supine lying receiver's hip.

Leave some space between your knee and receiver's body to allow her to roll later in the spinal twist.

Prep: Pick up receiver's closer leg and bring the bent knee up over receiver's hip into the vertical angle.

Thread your leg under receiver's bent knee and place your foot on the other side of her straight leg at the level of the knee.

With this move you are holding receiver's bent leg at the back of the knee in a lock over the other leg.

Exercise: Grab receiver's opposite arm with one hand and pull her into a spinal twist.

Place your other hand over her shoulder.

Release receiver's hand across her upper body to reach over to her raised shoulder now with both hands.

Hold the shoulder with your hand closer to receiver's head and start moving your other hand lower following the back side of the ribcage.

Pull receiver's upper body from your upper body weight over your hands and arms to enforce the spinal twist at each position on receiver's back all the way down to the hip and back to the shoulder again.

Rec: This exercise highly complicated but once you learn how to use your body properly you'll love this spinal twist.

Bm: Sitting and springing from your bent leg underneath you is the key for this exercise.

Also pay attention to your back and keep it straight as well as your arms.

Hints: Look for receiver holding her neck and head up.

Let her relax it and then continue with the stretch.

Sen Line: *Multiple*

Repeat from 3.1 to 3.25.5 with the other leg!

Chapter 3
Double leg exercises

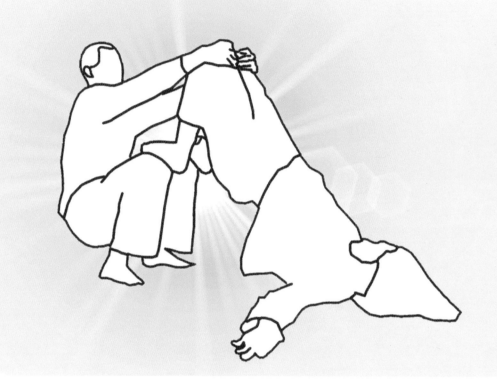

The double leg exercises designed to work with the hips and what connected to them, the legs and the torso, therefore they require strength and straight forward moves. Working with both legs at the same time can be challenging for your back. Please be careful and pay attention to your own body posture and body mechanics.

Ask receiver to put her arms over her head and remove the pillow from under receiver's head.

10 minutes of double leg work changes the dynamics of the lower and upper body.

4. Double leg exercises

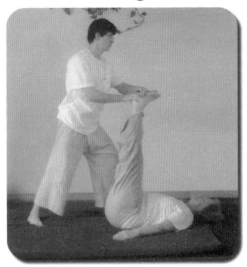

4.1 L-V-L

PP: Stand by receiver's legs on the side.

Prep: Lift up receiver's legs and hold them at the heels.

Exercise: Push both legs up to the vertical angle keeping them straight.

This is the "L" position. The name of the similar yoga pose is Viparita Karani.

From here push legs toward receiver's head to stretch receiver's posterior side until the hips starting to come up from the floor.

This is the "V" position. Then release and move back to the starting "L" position. Repeat it until receiver relaxes and ready for the next exercise.

Rec: Do not push the legs over the head.

Bm: When you get to the "L" position open your legs into a small Tai Chi like stand to be able to push from your legs and hip rather than from your upper body or arms.

Eff: This exercise is a warm up for the rest of the double leg exercises so do it gently.

Hints: It's a great exercise for receivers with stiff back and legs.

Sen Line: *Sen Sumana*

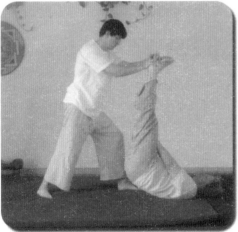

4.2 Push raised leg forward with counterpress on thighs above the knee

PP: Standing and holding receiver's legs in "L" or Viparita Karani position.

Prep: Keep receiver in "L" position and ask to place her hands on her thigh above her knees and lock her elbows straight.

Exercise: Push legs toward receiver's head.

You will feel the counterforce that receiver hold against your push. As you push harder the balance of your push and the counterforce will lift receiver's hip and lower back off of the floor. Continue the push until receiver's lower back fully comes up from the floor.

Then without holding it release it back to the "L" position.

Repeat it as many times you need.

Eff: The force and counterforce allow the hip, the spine and the lower back extend and stretch in a balanced and safe way.

Sen Line: *Sen Sumana*

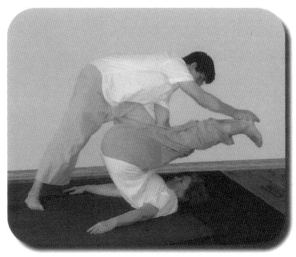

4.3 Assisted plough pose

PP: Again start from "L" position and open your legs into a rather big stance.
Prep: Place both hands on receiver's heels.
Exercise: Push receiver's legs all the way this time over her head.
Do it rather slowly to be able to sense the stretch and the flexibility of receiver.
If receiver able to touch her toes on the floor over her head you can hold both ankles with your inside hand and provide stability and support on her knees with your outside hand. Then release legs back to the "L" position.

Ci: Spinal injury, lower back surgery, ruptured disks are contraindicated.
Rec: Do this exercise once in a session. Do not repeat it.
Eff: This exercise is one of the greatest stretch for the posterior side of the body in our session.
Hints: Communicate with receiver and look for shaking in the leg and facial expression.
Sen Line: *Sen Sumana*

4.4 Knee to chest

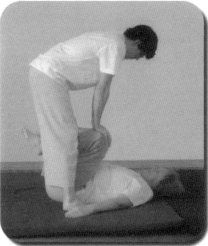

PP: Strating from the "L" position.
Prep: Bend receiver's both legs.
Push receiver's knees with both hands so the knees closing on the chest. If receiver is heavy or very stiff you can use your knees to stabilize the position and push her legs with your knees and hands together toward her chest. If the receiver rather flexible let receiver's feet hanging while holding her knees with your hands and walk up toward her shoulders pushing her knees forward between your legs as you are moving forward.
Exercise: With this move receiver's knees getting closer to her chest and some stretch starts to build up in the lower back and posterior side of her legs. In this position secure receiver's legs with your knees by pressing them gently together. Place your hands on receiver's knees and apply firm pressure.
Hold the stretch for about 5 seconds and then release.

Ci: Pregnancy, intestinal obstruction, hernia
Rec: The applied pressure on the knees can be in direction to the floor or direction away from receiver's body.
Eff: This exercise will lenghten receiver's lower back.
Sen Line: *Sen Sumana*

4.5 Lower back release

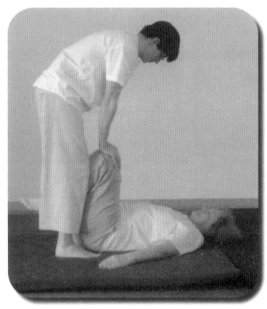

PP: Stand by receiver's bent legs.

Prep: Bring receiver's bend knees into the 90 degrees angle.

Support receiver's bend knees with your knees from the sides with pressing them gently.

Exercise: Apply firm pressure on her knees straight down toward the floor.

There is little or no movement at all so you just keep pressing for about 5 seconds.

Then release the pressure and apply it again but this time alternate between the two knees.

This time you will sens settle or bigger moves within the hip that massages the Sacroiliac joint.

Rec: Include this exercises in all of your sessions!

Eff: One of the greatest release for the lower back and consequently for the whole body.

Hints: Which hip is stiffer? Which sdie has more movement?

Sen Line: *Sen Sumana*

4.6 Knee circles

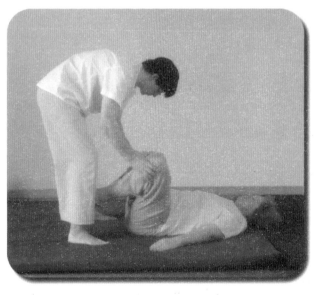

PP: Stand by receiver's legs in a bigger stance.

Prep: Lift up receiver's bent legs to the 90 degrees angle and hold them with your hands.

Exercise: Slowly start circle the knees around the hip.

Apply gentle pressure to make sure the knees stay together.

After several rounds change direction and rotate the knees to the opposite direction.

Rec: Lovely exercise recommended for every receivers.

Eff: Great exercise toward releasing and identifying hoding patterns of the leg, hip and abdomen.

Hints: Look for twitching, holding, jumping in the hip.

You'll be able to identify locked, blocked areas along the leg and abdomen.

Sen Line: *Multiple*

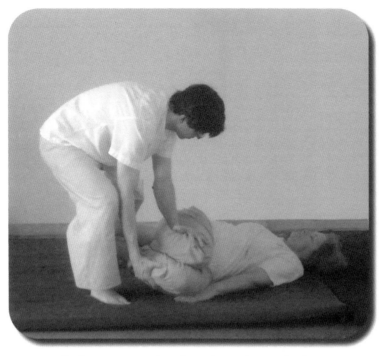

4.7 Spinal Twist double leg style

PP: Stand by receiver's legs in a rather big stance.

Prep: Lift up receiver's bent legs to the 90 degrees angle and hold them with your hands.

Exercise: This time to make sure the knees stay together apply firm or strong pressure on the sides of receiver's knees.

Step out to one side and move receiver's knees with you all the way turning receiver's spine.

Most receiver's will be able to go all the way to the floor but if you feel resistance during the twist stabilize the position.

After a short holding turn knees back to the starting position and repeat the twist to the other side.

Rec: This is a great way to do the spinaltwist.

Bm: Be strong and straight forward with this exercise!

Holding the legs together requires strenght.

You may use your weighted front leg passively to hold receiver's feet .

Hints: You'll probably find the sides different from each other as most receivers have quite a different flexibility on left and right.

Sen Line: *Multiple*

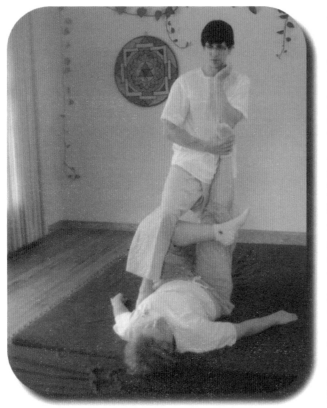

4.8 Vertical half lotus

PP: Stand by receiver's legs in the "L" position.

Prep: From the "L" Position bend one of receiver's knee and place the bend leg over straight leg so the ankle of the bent leg resting over straight leg.

Hold straight leg up.

Step over bent leg and place your foot by receiver's hip so you are supporting receiver's bend leg with the back of your leg.

Exercise: With a gentle tai chi move, move back and forth several times to stretch the straight leg and the lower back.

Then lock receiver's legs by moving and turning the straight leg front of you to brace it with your hip and thigh.

This lock gives you a stable stand and receiver will feel safe and supported.

Support the foot of the straight leg form underneath with your inside hand and roll the forearm of your outside arm on the sole of receiver's foot.

After this warm up, press your elbow into the six points of the sole.

When you release the elbow press extend your forearm straight forward for additional stretch.

You can also elbow press any known reflexology point of the sole.

Repeat the sequence on the other leg.

Ci: If you can't lock receiver's leg don't do not proceed to the elbow press.

Rec: If you haven't done Thai Chi before it's time to start.

Eff: This exercise gives great posterior side stretch with the combination of the movement of tai chi and reflexology work.

Hints: It can be painfull to hold the bent leg across the straight leg for receiver.

If this happens skip the exercise.

Sen Line: *Multiple*

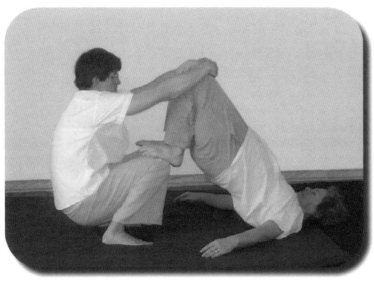

4.9 Assisted half bridge

PP: Stand by receiver's feet in supine position.

Prep: Lift both legs up and bend them into the Knees to chest position.

Place receiver's feet on your knees and open your stance (feet) apart with your toes pointing to the outside, so your lower legs forming a strong triangle.

Interlaced your fingers over receiver's knees.

Exercise: This exercises consists 2 dynamically different phases and it is one of the rare moment when you need activity from receiver.

In Phase 1 you want to pull receiver up from the floor.

It usually isn't an easy thing to accomplish so ask receiver to lift her hip up in the air.

Now you are ready for Phase 2 which is the stretch itself.

Slowly squat down and pull receiver's knees with you.

Hold it for a little while to allow receiver relax in this strange position.

Then release and place receiver back on the floor by coming up into the starting position.

Rec: Be careful as your knees can be sharp because of the bony patella and other knee features. It can be sensationfull for receiver especially with sensitive reflex points in the sole.

Bm: Keep in mind this time you need receiver's help.

You need to be very stable to able to hold up and balance receiver's weight.

The only way you can do it is forming a stable triangle with your legs. This position also called the duck squatting.

Eff: This exercise gives a great anterior stretch and also effect reflexology points of the foot.

It is also an inverted posture and great for enhancing circulation.

Hints: Hold your hands strongly together not allowing the knees to open.

Sen Line: *Sen Sumana*

4.10 Lifting with straight legs

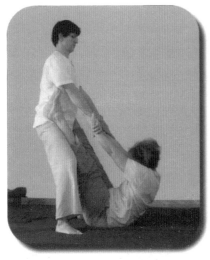

PP: Stand by receiver in "L" position.

Prep: Pick up receiver's straight legs and place it front of you.

Open receiver's leg a bit to reach down and ask her to hold on your forearm and you hold her forearm also.

Exercise: Squat down to allow yourself to make the pull from your leg not from your back and pull receiver up from the floor.

Then release her back to the starting position.

Repeat it 3 times.

You can go all the way to a slight back bend gradually.

Rec: You probably find this exercise different with each receivers depends on their height and leg length.

If the receiver is shorter than you keep her legs between your arms or slightly open.

Otherwise keep receiver's legs open and support them with your thighs.

Bm: Use your legs and not your back to pull receiver up!

Hints: Find the proper stand for yourself based on your receiver's height.

Sen Line: *Sen Sumana*

4.11 Lifting with crossed legs

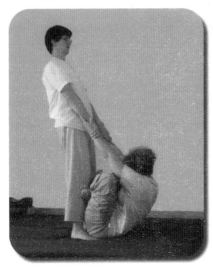

PP: Stand by receiver in "L" position.

Prep: From "L" position bend receiver's both leg to put them in the crossed formation and support the crossed legs with your lower legs.

Reach down and ask her to hold on your forearm and hold her forearm as well.

Exercise: Pull receiver up 3 times using your legs.

Rec: Again, increase the stertch gradually by leaning back more at each time of pull.

Bm: Bend your legs to initiate the pull from your legs and not from your back.

Sen Line: *Sen Sumana*

4.12 Lifting into sitting

PP: Hold receiver in the crossed leg position holding her legs with your lower legs.

Exercise: Pull up receiver as you did it before but this time step aside and tip receiver into sitting position.

Rec: This is a transition move from supine to sitting position that makes your session flowing.

Chapter 4
Upper body massage
Abdomen, chest, arms, hands head and face

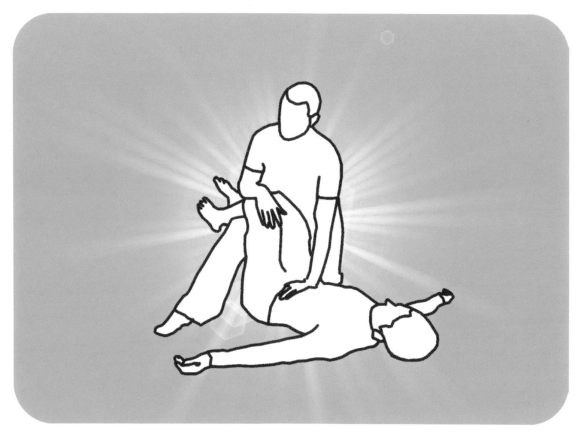

This chapter introduces a full sequence of exercises for the front upper body. Therapists will learn to apply simple and powerful techniques to give an effective massage focusing on the micro areas - the hands, face and the ears- of the body. These techniques can easily be incorporated into existing practice.

The main feature of this part of the session is the breathing. It is crucial to sense and follow the rhythm of receiver's breathing during exercises of the abdomen and the ribcage.

It is an easy to learn sequence with great features that missing from other modalities such as abdomen and arm massage. 15-20 minutes makes a good upper body massage.

5. Abdomen

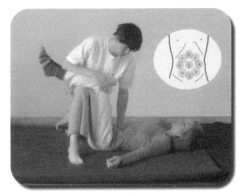

5.1 Palming abdomen in circle(E)

PP: Half kneel by receiver's hip.
Lift both of her legs up on top of your bent leg.
Prep: Place your inside arm on receiver's lower legs and knees.
In this position you're stable and fully supporting receiver that allows you to work with the relaxed abdomen. Alternatively you can use a pillow or bolster to elevate and bend receiver's legs. Stay in this position until the massage of the arms. We look at the abdomen area as circle or a wheel. It has 9 zones, 1 in the middle at the navel and 8 around it approximately equal distance and in size from the navel.
Exercise: Palm the abdomen starting at the navel and go to Point 2 to follow a counter clockwise direction to get to Point 2 again and back to the navel.
Palm once in each zone with the rhythm of receiver's breathing.
Ci: Pregnancy, recent abdominal surgery contraindicates any kind of abdominal work.
Rec: The palming of the abdominal area should be gentle and relaxing.
Eff: The main effect is the relaxation of the belly.
The counter clockwise direction is slows down the intestinal traffic. If you do the palming with clockwise direction you will speed things up.
It is good in case of constipation but not such a good thing for receiver with regular digestive and eliminating activity.
Hints: Remember this area can hold lots of tension and is the center of emotions.
Sen Line: *Multiple*

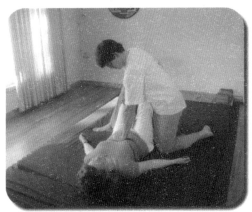

5.2 Deep palming in nine zones(E)

PP: Half kneeling by receiver's hip with both of receiver's legs up on top of your bent leg.
Prep: The nine zones are the same for deep palming.
Exercise: Start at the navel again but this time apply different pressure and timing.
Palm press the navel on receiver's exhale and keep it pressed through the upcoming inhale to press deeper and direction toward the navel with the next exhale then release.
Move to the next zone and repeat the deep press.
Go around the zones with this technique to get back to the navel.

Ci: Pregnancy, recent abdominal surgery contraindicates any kind of abdominal work. Intestinal obstruction is also contraindication.

Hints: You'll feel the solar plexus and the arteries pumping blood under the intestinal track. It is ok to sense this energy but do not block it with too much pressure.

Sen Line: *Multiple*

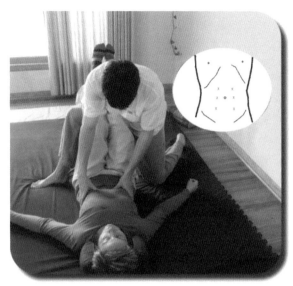

5.3 Deep thumb press six points

PP: Half kneeling by receiver's hip with both of receiver's legs up on top of your bent leg.

Prep: The points are equal distance from the navel which is it about 1 thumb length. It is the length of receiver's thumb, not yours.

There are 2 points superior to the navel on each side, next 2 points are in level with the navel on each side and the last 2 points are inferior to the navel on each side.

Exercise: Thumb press the 2 points on the same level with both thumbs in the same time.

Starting at the 2 points on top.

Then move to the next 2 points and down to the lowest 2 points and come all the way back the same way to the top 2 points.

Ci: Pregnancy, recent abdominal surgery contraindicates any kind of abdominal work. Intestinal obstruction is also contraindication.

Rec: Press each point on exhale only and release them with the upcoming inhale.

Sen Line: *Sen Ittha-Pingkhala*

Repeat Exercise 5.1 Palming abdomen in circle (E)!

6. Chest

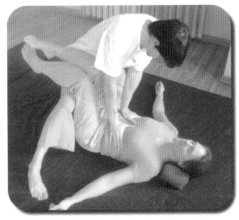

6.1 Double palm press ribcage

PP: Half kneeling by receiver's hip with both of receiver's legs up on top of your bent leg.

Prep: Place your palms with thumbs open on receiver's lower ribcage.

Exercise: Palm press on exhale down and away from head to lengthen receiver's front upper body then release with the inhale.

Move your hands up higher on ribcage and repeat the palm press then move back to first position and repeat palm press again.

Rec: Be respectfull with woman doing this exercise.

Stay under the bra line or ask for permission.

Do not press on breasts!

Eff: It is a great exercise to facilitate full breathing cycle and great stretch for the whole upper body.

Sen Line: *Multiple*

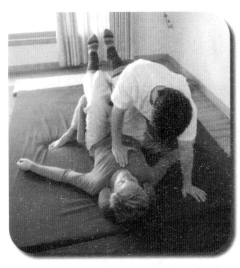

6.2 Single palmpress sternum(E)

PP: Half kneeling by receiver's hip with both of receiver's legs up on top of your bent leg.

Prep: Place one hand on the floor in the area aside receiver's shoulder for balancing your weight.

Place your other palm on distal end of receiver's sternum.

Exercise: Palm press sternum from above the Xiphoid process all the way up and back following receiver's breathing pattern.

Use your balancing hand on the floor to create lenghtening effect on receiver's chest as you palm press not only downward but away from receiver's head.

Rec: Plam press firmly and gradually.

Eff: This is one of the best breathing facilitator exercises.

Hints: Stay away from breast tissue for woman!

Sen Line: *Sen Sumana*

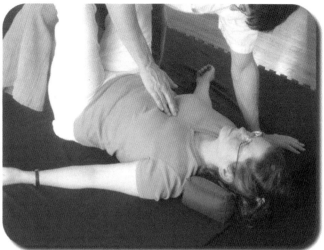

6.3 3 fingers circle sternum(E)

PP: Half kneeling by receiver's hip with both of receiver's legs up on top of your bent leg.
Prep: Place one hand on the floor in the area aside receiver's shoulder for balancing your weight.
Place your 3 middle fingers on distal end of receiver's sternum.
Exercise: Slowly and firmly press and optionally circle the 3 fingers up and down the sternum.
Sen Line: *Multiple*

Repeat Exercise 6.2 Single palm press sternum (E)!

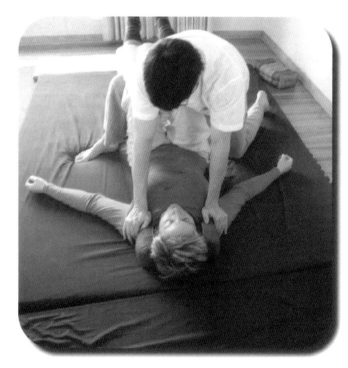

6.4 Double palm press shoulders(E)

PP: Half kneeling by receiver's hip with both of receiver's legs up on top of your bent leg.
Prep: Place your palms on receiver's shoulders.
Exercise: Press both shoulders down and hold it for a little while then release.
Sen Line: *Sen Kalathari*

7. Arms and hands

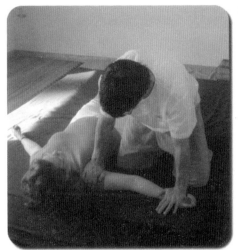

7.1 Arm stretch to the side(E)

PP: Kneel beside receiver's upper body at her dominant side.
Prep: Pull receiver's arm to a 90 degrees angle to the side.
Place your hands on receiver's wrist and shoulder.
Exercise: Palm press both end of receiver's arm in the same time.
Rather lengthening than pressing into the floor.
Sen Line: *Multiple*

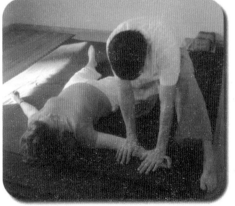

7.2 Palming the medial arm(E)

PP: Come up to half kneeling beside receiver's upper body at her dominant side.
Prep: Place your hands on receiver's wrist and shoulder.
Exercise: Palm from receiver's wrist and shoulder to her elbow and back, then turn and palm back to the elbow again and finish palming down on the forearm to the wrist. This palming pattern is the same as you did before on the legs warming up for the Energy Line work.
Sen Line: *Multiple*

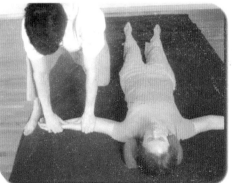

7.3 Thumbing medial arm(E)

PP: Half kneeling beside receiver's upper body at her dominant side.
Prep: Place your thumbs on receiver's middle Energy Line at the wrist.
Exercise: Thumb press the middle Energy Line from wrist to elbow and back.
Then palm your way up to the upper arm and thumb press the upper arm from elbow to shoulder and back.

Finish with stretching receiver's arm with palm press at the wrist and at the shoulder.
Sen Line: *Sen Kalathari*

Repeat Exercise 7.2 Palming the medial arm(E)!

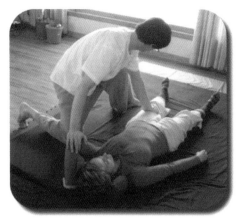

7.4 Stretch bent arm away (E)

PP: Half kneeling by the side of receiver.
Prep: Bend her arm and place her hand by her ear creating a triangle.
Place one hand on the top of this triangle on her elbow and place your other hand on receiver's thigh on the same side.
Exercise: Push your hands away to stretch and lengthen receiver's shoulder, upper body, and hip. Repeat the stretch as many times as you need with changing your hand position on the thigh.
Ci: Don't do this exercise if receiver not able to turn her hand toward her shoulder.
Rec: This exercise creates a great stretch and is very likeable.
Bm: Place receiver's hand pointing toward her shoulder to prevent strain on the wrist.
Eff: Creates a great stretch on the side of the body.
Hints: Make sure receiver's bent arm is relaxed.
Sen Line: *Sen Sahatsarangsi-Thawari*

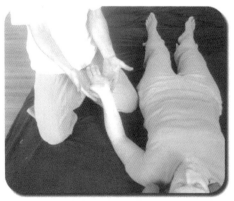

7.5 Squeez hand

PP: Sitting beside receiver.
Prep: Hold receiver's hand with both hands with dorsal surface up.
Exercise: Squeez it by pulling your hands apart.
Eff: It warms up receivers hand.
Sen Line: *Multiple*

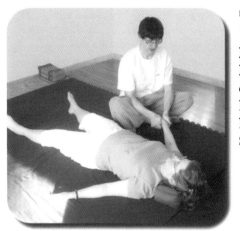

7.6 Hand lock

PP: Sitting or kneeling.
Prep: Turn receiver's hand palmar surface up and slide your little fingers between the thumb and index finger and between the ring and little fingers. Open your hands to stretch and support receiver's hand.
Eff: This way the whole palmar surface of the hand is available for your thumbs to work with.
Sen Line: *Multiple*

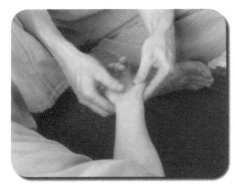

7.7 Strokes with thumbs

PP: Sitting or kneeling.
Prep: Hold receiver's hand in the lock.
Exercise: Make strokes with your thumbs on the outer parts of the palm toward the thumb and the little finger. You can do the strokes simultaneously or alternated.
Rec: This is one of the greatest feeling for receiver of the whole session so do it every time.
Sen Line: *Sen Sumana, multiple*

7.8 Thumbing palmar surface

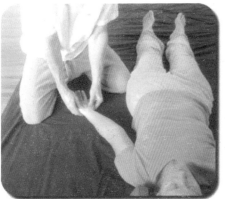

PP: Sitting or kneeling.
Prep: Hold receiver's hand in the lock.
Exercise: Thumb the palmar surface from the middle point of the palm close to the wrist with both of your thumbs in the same time with one thumb going toward receiver's little finger other thumb going to the thumb. Before you reach the MP joint change thumbing to circular movement and circle all the way to the fingertips.
Thumb again from the starting point toward the ring and index fingers the same way. And for last thumb from the starting point toward the middle finger.
Hints: Look for artrithis and swollen joints.Also cuts and minor injuries can be unpleseant to press or stroke on.
Sen Line: *Sen Kalathari*

7.9 Thumb circles on dorsal surface

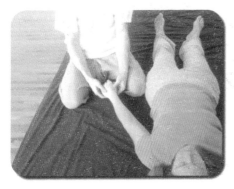

PP: Sitting or kneeling.
Prep: Hold receiver's hand with both hands, palm down.
Exercise: Start with a firm press on the middle point of the hand close to the wrist. Then thumb circle with both thumbs simultaneously toward the fingers all the way to the tip of the fingers, first to the thumb and little finger then toward the index and ring fingers and finish with the middle finger.
Rec: Very good exercise for receiver with joint pain or disease such as arthritis.
Sen Line: *Sen Kalathari*

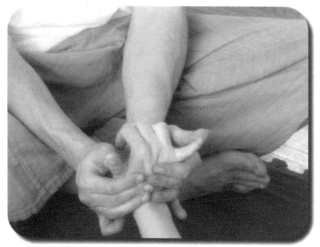

7.10 Glide and stretch fingers

PP: Sitting or kneeling
Prep: Hold receiver's hand with your fingers on the dorsal surface and your thumbs on the palmar surface.
Exercise: Slowly glide your thumbs on the palm toward the fingers and stretch the fingers as you approach the tips.
Do it with the same finger selection as you did previously:
Thumb and little finger first, then the index and ring fingers and finish with the middle finger.
Sen Line: *Sen Kalathari*

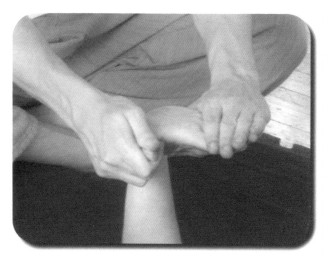

7.11 Wrist stretch

PP: Sitting or kneeling.
Prep: Turn receiver's hand palm up resting on her elbow.
Exercise: Stretch the fingers away from the thumb by pushing them toward the floor so the palm will open nicely facing to the ceiling.
Rec: Include this stretch in your sessions.
Eff: It is a great stretch not only for the hand but for the whole arm.
Sen Line: *Sen Kalathari*

Repeat from Exercise 7.1 to 7.11 with other arm and hand!

8.1 Head and face massage(E)

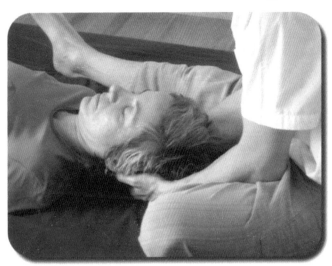

PP: Sit or kneel by the top of receiver's head.

Prep: Palm the shoulders toward the neck to connect the energy from the arms .

Exercise: Finger circle the back of the neck several times up and down.

Place and touch your fingers under receiver's neck with thumbs up.

Lift your fingers and receiver's neck upward with outward rolling move from C7 all the way up to the occiput.

Hook your 3 middle fingers on each side under receiver's skull and hold it for 10-20 seconds.

Release the holding and hold receiver's head with your fingers from underneath so your fingers covering the middle line of her head.

Slowly change hand position toward the top of the head by rolling the head to the sides.

When you reach the top of the head place it on the floor and place your thumbs on the Crown Chakra.

Slowly walk your thumbs to the hairline and to the 3rd Eye and place your thumbs on the 3rd Eye.

From the 3rd Eye make strokes toward the temple on the forehead 3-4 times up to the hairline.

Follow the Energy Lines under the eyes place your fingers close to the nose and follow the geography of the cheek bones toward the sides.

Underneath the nose pull your thumbs apart to the sides.

Repeat this move under the mouth on the chin.

Finish the facemassage with rubbing the jaw between your fingers and thumbs all the way up to the ears.

Massage the ears gently then cover them for 30 seconds with your cuphands.

Rec: You can freestyle this part of the session by adding your bag of tricks from different modalities.

Eff: These strokes relax and syncronize the mind with the body.

Sen Line: *Multiple*

Chapter 5
Side position

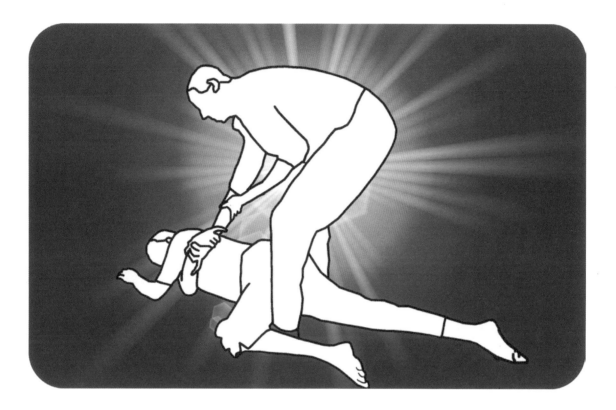

The side position is probably the greatest part of Thai massage. It is one of the favorite both of receivers and therapists.

First of all it is a very comfortable body position for receiver. The side position allows therapist to perform the whole 2 hour session which means a lot for pregnant women and receivers with lower back pain or other conditions which restrict them to be in the supine position for prolonged time during the session.

Side position also gives a unique access to the body to perform precise work with the shoulders and back. Therapists can top this part of the session with great, full body stretches. Spend enough time in side position at least 15 minutes each sides!

9. Side position

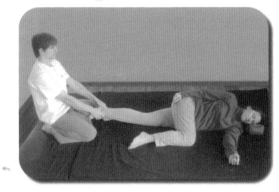

9.1 Pull straight leg

PP: Kneel by the foot of receiver's straight leg.
Prep: Grab the ankle with both hands.
Pull it firmly to straight the whole body to align the spine and hip.
Make sure the bent leg is in 90 degrees angle with the straight leg and the hip is somewhat vertical.

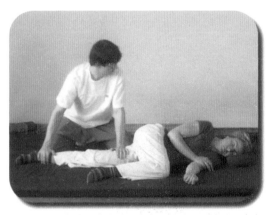

9.2 Palming inside straight leg

PP: Kneel or half kneel by the side of receiver's straight leg in level with the knee to be able to reach equally to the thigh and to the ankle.
Exercise: Start palming from the ankle and from the proximal end of the thigh toward the knee and back then back to the knee to conclude the palming at the ankle.
Sen Line: *Sen Sumana*

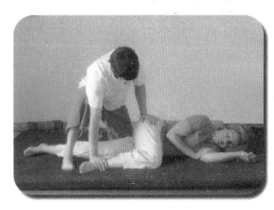

9.3 Palming bent leg(E)

PP: Half kneel across receiver's straight leg and place your front foot by the foot of receiver's bent leg.
Prep: Place your hands on the heel and the hip of receiver's bent leg.
Exercise: Palm toward the knee and back then to the knee again to finish up at the ankle again.
Sen Line: *Sen Ittha-Pingkhala*

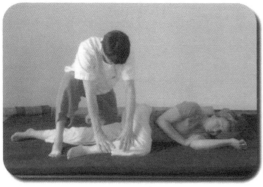

9.4.1 Thumbing lower bent leg(E)

PP: Half kneel across receiver's straight leg.

Prep: The 3rd outside Energy Line of the leg runs up on the lateral side of the foot and connects up to the head of the fibula.

From here it passes the knee on the side and follows the posterior edge of the IT band.

At hip level the line covers the glutes in a boomerang shape and runs to the front of the hip.

Exercise: Start thumbing the 3rd outside Energy Line from the ankle to the knee and back to the ankle again.

Palm the lower leg again to connect up to the thigh.

Bm: The change of kneeling between the lower leg and the thigh is crucial.

Sen Line: *Sen Ittha-Pingkhala*

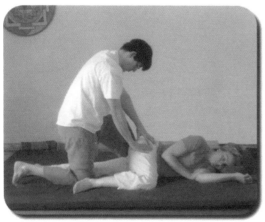

9.4.2 Thumbing upper bent leg and boomerang(E)

PP: Half kneel facing toward receiver with your inside knee between receiver's legs and your outside foot behind receiver's back.

If you're transitioning from the previous exercise change your knees on the floor.

Exercise: Continue thumbing the 3rd outside Energy Line of the thigh from the knee to the hip and back to the knee following the groove between the IT band, Vastus lateralis and the hamstring group.

Palm up to the hip and palm around it following the boomerang.

Thumb the boomerang around the hip several times.

Rec: Thumb around the Greater trochanter and feel the different tones of the tissues.

Spend some times at several points along the boomerang.

Eff: Relaxes and soothes the deep lateral rotators and the other components of the Trochanteric Fan.

Hints: The Throcanteric Fan is Thomas Myers' description of the region of the Greater trochanter and the components attaching to it.

Sen Line: *Sen Ittha-Pingkhala*

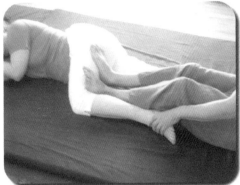

9.5 Flipped grape press

PP: Sit between receiver's legs.
Prep: Place your feet on posterior side of receiver's thigh behind the knee.
Exercise: Press the entire posterior side of receiver's thigh with your inside foot moving up and down between the knee and the Ischial Tuberosity.
Rec: Use this exercise when you enconter stiffness or pain during thumbing.
Bm: Adjust your seat to optimize your foot pressure.
Hints: Keep receiver's knee from sliding on the floor.
That would ruin the exercise.
Sen Line: *Sen Ittha-Pingkhala*

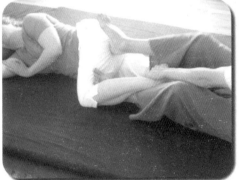

9.6 Twisted wine (leg locked for support)

PP: Sit between receiver's legs.
Prep: Place your outside foot behind receiver's bent knee on the back of the thigh and bring receiver's bent lower leg across your leg into a lock.
Place your inside foot on receiver's bent leg behind the knee on the 3rd outside line.
Exercise: Press your heel deep into the line and hold it for 5 seconds on each point as you moving toward the hip and then back to the knee.
Rec: You can reach the boomerang that you can explore with your heel gently.
Sen Line: *Sen Ittha-Pingkhala*

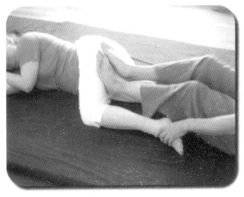

9.7 Flipped double grape press

PP: Sit between receiver's legs.
Prep: Release the lock if you transitioning from previous exercise.
Place both of your feet on receiver's bent leg on the thigh behind the knee.
Exercise: Walk with both feet on the back of receiver's thigh between the knee and the hip.
Sen Line: *Sen Ittha-Pingkhala*

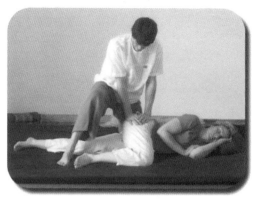

9.8 Palming boomerang(E)

PP: Kneel or half kneel behind receiver in level with her hips.
Exercise: Palm the hip following the boomerang with both hands.
Rec: You can palm with palm on palm or use alternated palming.
Sen Line: *Sen Ittha-Pingkhala*

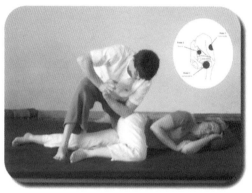

9.9 Elbow press boomerang points(E)

PP: Kneel or half kneel behind receiver in level with her hips.
Prep: The *1st point* of the boomerang is located between the Greater Trhochater and the Ischial Tuberosity.
The *2nd point* located over the periformis muscle close to the attachment with the Femur.
The *3rd point* is located over the Gluteus Medius and Minimus muscle half way between the Iliac Crest and the Femur.
Exercise: You have 2 options here.
Option 1 is using your thumbs to press the points and palm each point after thumb press.
Option 2 is using your elbows pressing the points and palm each point after elbow press.
With the elbow *Point 1* is doable with your elbow closer to receiver's head.
Points 2 and 3 more accessible with elbow closer to receiver's feet.
To make sure your pressure is firm and not too sharp use your other hand and arm like a triangle to create the pressure over the other elbow on the point.
Rec: These points can be highly sensitive especially *Point 2*.
For locating the points use your thumbs and be creative with your elbows.
Bm: For the optimal pressure use your upper body through your other arm for the elbow press.
Hints: These points are represented by physical structures.
Point 1 is involves Quatratus femoris and Obturator externus, *Point 2* is matches with Piriformis and *Point 3* is a crucial point of tension of Gluteus Medius and Minimus.
Sen Line: *Sen Ittha-Pingkhala*

Repeat Exercise 9.8 Palming boomerang(E)!

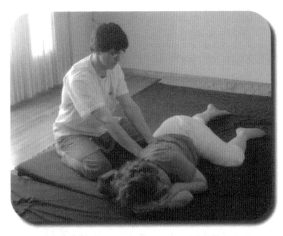

9.10 Palming back lines(E)

PP: Kneel behind receiver's back in level with her lower back.

Exercise: Double palm the entire back above the spine from the sacrum up to T4, T5 between the scapulas and back.

You can also alternate the palming to walk up and down the back.

Sen Line: *Multiple*

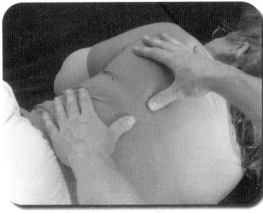

9.11 Thumbing back lines(E)

PP: Kneel behind receiver's back in level with her lower back.

Prep: *Line 2* runs along the spine in the groove between the erectors and the spine.

Line 3 runs on the top of the ridge of the erector group.

Line 4 runs from the top of the iliac crest to the lower corner of the scapula.

Exercise: Thumb *Line 2,3,* up and down from the hip up to T4 T5 between the scapulas and back.

Thumb *Line 4* only to the lower corner of the scapula and back.

Rec: Techniques for *Line 1* will be introduce later as part of advanced training.

Sen Line: *Multiple*

Repeat Exercise 9.10 Palming back lines(E)!

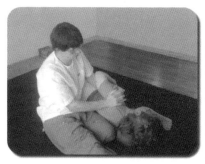

9.12 Shoulder circles

PP: Kneel parallel behind receiver.
Prep: Straight out your outside leg and sit on the ankle of your bent inside leg.
This sitting feel strange at first but it going to be very comfy and stable to work with the shoulder and neck.
Lift up receiver's top arm and swim your hand under it to reach to the front covering the front of the shoulder.
With your outside hand reach ahead and interlace your fingers on receiver's shoulder.
Exercise: Brace the shoulder with your palms and rotate it around several times forward and backward.
Rec: These rotations should be done rather slow to be able to assess the condition of the shoulder.
Bm: Hold receiver's top arm by resting it on the top of your inside lower arm while rotating the shoulder.
Sen Line: *Multiple*

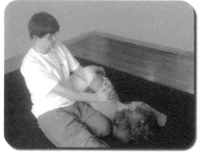

9.13 Shoulder and neck stretch

PP: Paralell kneeling behind receiver with straight outside leg and bent inside leg.
Prep: Hold receiver's shoulder with your inside hand on the front from underneath receiver's top arm.
Exercise: Interlace your fingers on top of receiver's shoulder and pull it away from her head by leaning backward with your upper body.
Sen Line: *Sen Kalathari*

9.14 Shoulder and neck stretch with finger press

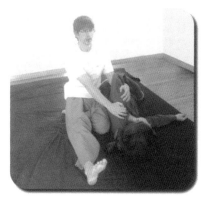

PP: Paralell kneeling behind receiver with straight outside leg and bent inside leg.
Prep: Hold receiver's shoulder with your inside hand on the front from underneath receiver's top arm.
Exercise: Place the fingers of your outside hand on the shoulder blade.
Pull the shoulder back with your inside arm and in the same time hook your fingers into the shoulder blade and pull with it too. Repeat this pull with changing your hooking fingers to different spots on the shoulder blade.
Rec: Great exercise for tense shoulders.
Sen Line: *Sen Kalathari*

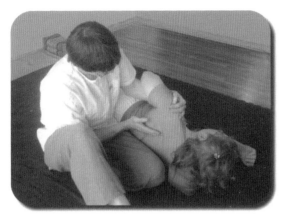

9.15 Palming with the blade of the palm around medial edge of scapula(E)

PP: Kneeling or sitting behind receiver's back.

Prep: Swim your inside hand between receiver's upper arm and upper body and place it on the front of receiver's shoulder.
Place the medial edge of your outside hand between receiver's scapula and spine.

Exercise: Press the edge of your palm into the place between the spine and scapula and pull the shoulder backward with your other hand in the same time.
Move up and down with this palm press around the medial edge of the scapula.

Rec: Check if you can get underneath the scapula with your palm at the lower portion.

Bm: The best position to do this is the crossed leg sitting when you can use your upper body and knee to lean in.

Eff: This exercise releases lots of tension and blockage around the mid back and effects the whole upper body structure.

Hints: Look for closeness and opennes of the scapula.

Sen Line: *Sen Kalathari*

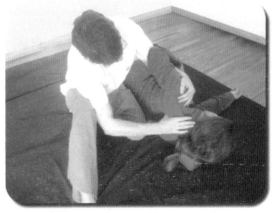

9.16 Thumbing around medial edge of scapula(E)

PP: Kneel or sit behind receiver's back

Prep: Slip your inside hand between receiver's upper arm and upper body and place it on the front of receiver's shoulder.

Exercise: Thumb around the medial edge of the scapula with the counter the force on the shoulder by pulling it with your other hand against your thumb.

Bm: Use your outside knee to hold and push your elbow to controll thumbing.

Hints: Look for ropy, tight, strap like muscle and fascia layers around and beneath the scapula.

Sen Line: *Sen Kalathari*

Repeat Exercise 9.15 Palming with the blade of the palm around medial edge of scapula(E)!

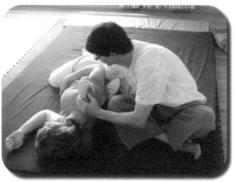

9.17 Stretch front upper body with pivot forearm leverage

PP: Kneel or sit behind receiver's back.

Prep: Slip your inside hand between receiver's upper arm and upper body and place it on the front of receiver's shoulder.

Interlace your fingers over receiver's shoulder.

Turn your inside forearm against receiver's back.

Exercise: Pull the shoulder back with both hands and push with your forearm against receiver's back to create a nice stretch over receiver's front upper body.

Repeat this stretch with changing the position of your forearm on the back between the hip and the scapula.

Rec: It isn't an essential exercise but I recommend to include your regular session as it gives great sensation to receiver.

Bm: Lean into the twist with your upper body.

Hints: Look for holding patterns.

Sen Line: *Sen Kalathari*

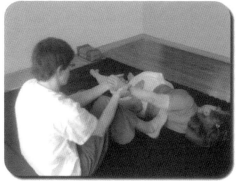

9.18 Arm stretch with rocking

PP: Sit behind receiver's back in level with her upper back facing toward receiver.

Prep: Pick up receiver's upper arm and stretch it back and hold it by the thumb and the wrist.

Place your feet on receiver's back one foot across her sacrum and the other foot by the scapulas.

Your foot over the sacrum will not touch the floor but the heel of your other foot will rest on the floor to support the back.

Exercise: Push first with the ball of your foot on the erector muscle group to roll receiver's body slightly forward with letting her arm and shoulder rolling forward too.

Then pull the arm back by leaning backward in your sitting while stabilizing the lower back with your other foot.

Repeat this rocking motion with changing your foot position following the erector muscle group between the sacrum and the scapulas.

Rec: This exercise holds the key body mechanics, rhythm and sync that crucial to perform a flowing balancing session.

Bm: Work from your core.

Eff: Opens and energizes the spine and the whole upper body.

Hints: Look for stiff shoulder, and potential pain in the front of the shoulder when stretching the arm backward.

Sen Line: *Sen Kalathari*

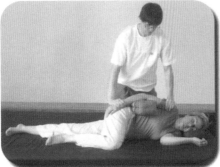

9.19 Palming lateral arm(E)

PP: Half kneeling behind receiver.
Prep: Place receiver's arm on top of the side of her body so her hand rests on her hip.
Exercise: Palm the arm from the wrist and from the shoulder toward the elbow and back and back to the elbow again then palm all the way down to the wrist.
Rec: Place a small pillow underneath the elbow to avoid discomfort or forcing receiver to hold her arm up.
Sen Line: *Multiple*

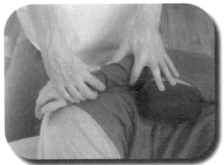

9.20 Thumbing lateral arm(E)

PP: Kneeling behind receiver.
Prep: The middle Energy Line runs in the middle of the forearm between the Radius and Ulna and continues over the Triceps all the way to the shoulder.
Exercise: Thumb-chasing-thumb from wrist to elbow and back on the middle Energy Line, then palm up to the elbow.
Thumb-chasing-thumb the upper arm following the middle Energy Line up to the shoulder and down.
Sen Line: *Sen Kalathari*

Repeat Exercise 9.19 Palming lateral arm(E)!

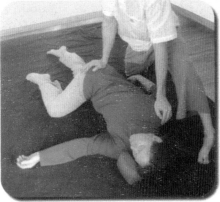

9.21 Gentle spinal twist(E)

PP: Half kneeling behind receiver in level with her hips.
Prep: Place your inside hand on the top of receiver's hip and your outside hand on receiver's shoulder.
Exercise: Gently push your hands with shoulder and hip away from each other to create a stretch and the spinal twist so the hip rotates to the front and the shoulder rotates to the back.
Repeat it several times.
You can adjust the leverage by changing your inside hand position on receiver's thigh up and down all the way to the knee and back.
Rec: This exercise is excellent for stiff people.
Bm: Utilize your upper body weight to push your hands apart.
Sen Line: *Multiple*

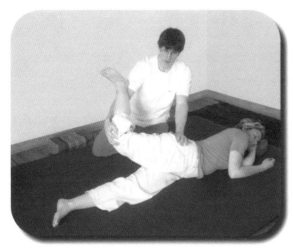

9.22.1 Bent leg stretch #1 with pivot hand (E)

PP: Kneeling behind receiver's straight leg.
Prep: This exercise made up of 4 steps to save your back and promote the flow of movements.
Exercise:
Step1: Pull the ankle of receiver's bent leg over her straight leg and place it just above the knee.
Step2: Pull the whole bent leg toward yourself holding it by the ankle and grab the lifting knee with your other hand.

Now you are holding receiver's bent leg by its knee with the lower leg and feet sticking out over your elbow.

Step3: Place your other hand on receiver's hip just under the iliac crest close to the sacrum and move yourself backward in a circular path all the way to the point of resistance of receiver's bent leg in your other hand.

Let receiver's hip slightly roll forward to allow hip open on the front rather than abducting the leg.

Step4: Lean on your arm resting on receiver's hip and pull the knee of the bent leg back in the same time to create a stretch across the front of receiver's body.

Hold the stretch for a while and place the leg back to its starting position on the floor.

Ci: Hernia

Bm: To create the stretch across the front of the body you need to make sure that you are not compressing the lower back.

Press the hip away from the upper body when you lean on your hand on receiver's hip and not toward the floor.

Eff: Opens the front of the body and stretches the deep layers of the psoas.

Sen Line: *Sen Sahatsarangsi-Thawari, Sen Sumana*

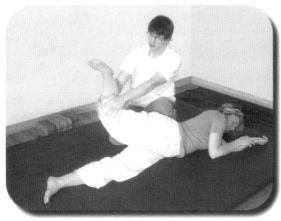

9.22.2 Bent leg stretch #2 with pivot knee

PP: Kneeling behind receiver's straight leg.
Prep: This exercise made up from 3 steps to save your back and promote the flow of movements.
Exercise:
Step1: Pull the ankle of receiver's bent leg over her straight leg apnd place it just above the knee.
Step2: Pull the whole bent leg toward yourself holding it by the ankle and grab the lifting knee with your other hand.
Now you are holding receiver's bent leg by its knee with the lower leg and feet sticking out over your elbow.
Step3: Place your closer knee to receiver's upper body on receiver's hip below the iliac crest close to the sacrum.
Place your other hand on receiver's bent leg and interlace your fingers over it.
Pull receiver's bent by leaning back and in the same time press on receiver's hip away from her upper body with your knee.
Rec: This exercise requiers great sense of balance and positioning.
Bm: Use your foot to drive your knee away from receivers body to lengthen the lower spine.
Sen Line: *Sen Sahatsarangsi-Thawari, Sen Sumana*

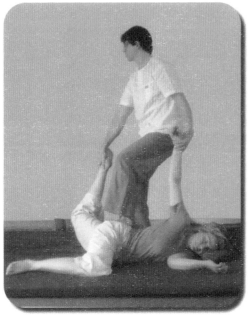

9.23 Straight leg stretch by the foot and hand

PP: Stand behind receiver.
Prep: Pick up receiver's straight leg by the ankle and slowly move backward in a circular path up to the point of resistance.
Ask for receiver's top arm and hold on to it only for balancing.
Don't pull or try to stretch it.
Place your closer foot to receiver's hip and balance yourself in this position.
Exercise: Turn your upper body away from receiver toward the side and gently press and lenghten receiver's hip and lower back.

Rec: You can find the point of resistance in a passive form in this exercise. Watch out for movement of the bent leg when you are stretching the staight leg .

Bm: You have to have a greate sense of balance for this exercise.

Eff: This turn will bring your arm to pull receiver's leg and thus creates a stretch across her body.

Sen Line: *Multiple*

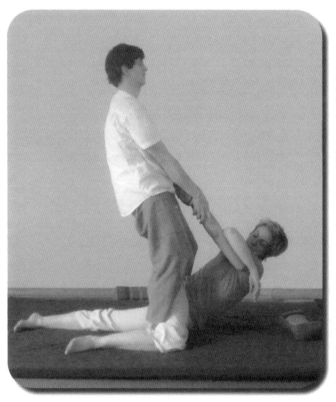

9.24 Spinal twist pull up style(E)

PP: Stand in a small open stand with receiver's straight leg between your feet.

Prep: Tuck one foot under receiver's bent leg just above the knee and support receiver's hip from behind with your other foot.

Ask receiver for her arm underneath and grab her wrist and also ask her to hold on yours.

Place receiver's other arm on top of the held arm.

Exercise: Bend your knees and pull receiver's arm up to bring the arm into greater angle.

Come up by straightening your legs and lean back to pull receiver's upper body up into a spinal twist. Great!

Ci: This exercise is contraindicated for receiver with lower back surgery or injury.

Rec: Always lift receiver from your legs and not from your back.

Not recommended with stiff, heavy receiver.

Bm: Use your legs to lift receiver up.

Sen Line: *Multiple*

Chapter 6
Back position

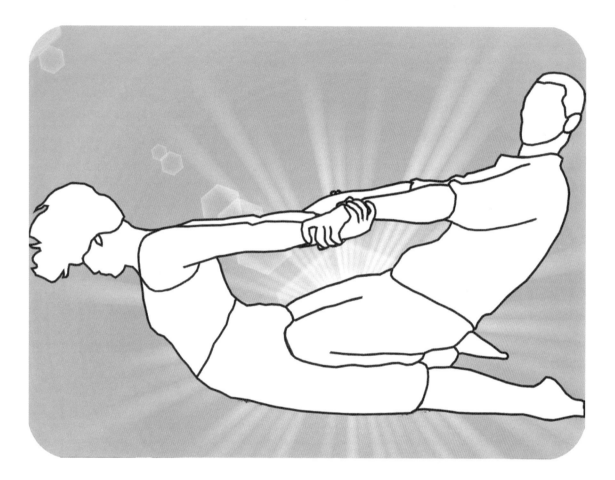

The back or prone position is very popular is western massage modalities. In Thai massage it features focused energy line work and great codependent positions.

Working in this position allows you to work with all the primary and secondary curves of the body which can make tremendous difference in energy flow and posture.

While the majority of the work is done on the back of the body, the front and the deep layers will be even more stretched and worked out.

Optimal time for the back position is 15 minutes.

10. Back position

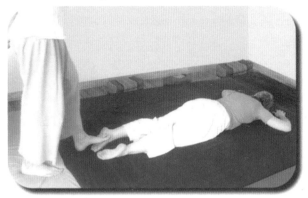

10.1 Foot massage with balls of the feet(E)

PP: Stand by receiver's feet facing toward her.

Exercise: Press the ball of your foot on receiver's sole. Cover the area between the ball of the foot and the heel. Start with one foot then repeat it on the other foot.

Rec: Receiver with stiff ankle are not good candidate for this exercise. They rather need a bolster underneath their ankles and you can work their soles with your knuckles instead.

Sen Line: *Sen Kalathari*

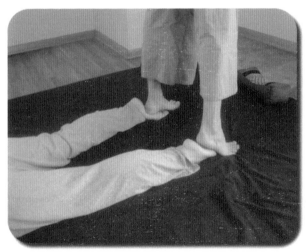

10.2 Foot massage with heels(E)

PP: Stand by receiver's feet backward, facing away from receiver.

Exercise: Press your heels on receiver's soles simultaneously or alternated.

Ci: Receiver with stiff ankle are not good candidate for this exercise.

Sen Line: *Sen Kalathari*

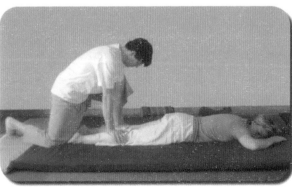

10.3 Palming posterior legs

PP: Half kneel between or across receiver's legs.

Exercise: Palm both legs up all the way to the Ischial Tuberosity and back down to the heel.

Use simultaneous palming.

Rec: Skip the back of the knees.

Double or simultaneous palming works better on the back side.

Sen Line: *Sen Sumana*

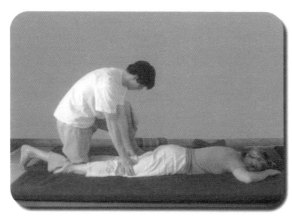

10.4 Thumbing posterior legs

PP: Half kneel between or across receiver's legs.

Exercise: Thumb the midline of the posterior leg simultaneously up and down the from the heel to the Iscial Tuberosity.

Rec: Skip the back of the knees.

Sen Line: *Sen Sumana*

Repeat Exercise 10.3 Palming posterior legs!

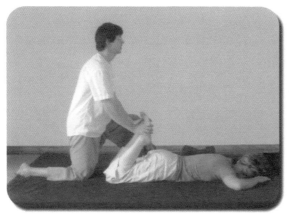

10.5 Heels to butt(E)

PP: Half kneel close to receiver's knees.

Prep: Bend receiver's legs by lifting the feet off of the floor.

Exercise: Grab the feet and cover the dorsal surface of receiver's feet with your hands.

Push them forward then release.

Don't hold the legs flexed too long rather assess the flexibility and range of motion of the leg.

Repeat this push several times with the variations from the Foot massage, 1.4, 1.5, 1.6.

Ci: Not recommended for receiver's with knee replacement.

Rec: Use your lunge stance to create the push from your hip rather than using your arm strength.

Sen Line: *Sen Kalathari*

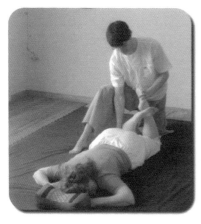

10.6 Heel to butt with crossed leg

PP: Half kneel close to receiver's knees.

Prep: Lift receiver's legs by the ankles and bend her legs at the knees.

Let receiver's leg fold on other leg behind the other knee. Hold on receiver's ankle that is still upright and place your other hand on folded leg's thigh.

Exercise: Push receiver's upright foot toward her butt and palm press the other thigh in the same time with the 1-2-3-2-1 pattern.

Sen Line: *Multiple*

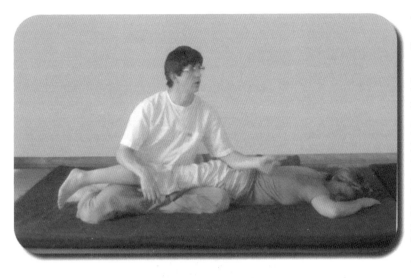

10.7 Teatime, Thai sitting(E)

PP: Sit between receiver's legs by her ankles facing away from her.

Prep: This exercise is a great example of the transition moves that makes your session flowing.

Turn to the side and lift up receiver's leg by the ankle.

Push the ankle high up and forward to create space under the leg for your thigh and slide your bent leg under receiver's upper thigh.

As close you can position your thigh to receiver's hip the better will be the outcome of this relaxing exercise.

Exercise: Now, you are in the thai sitting, receiver's straight leg front of your on your thighs.

Be creative with your forearms and elbows to press and roll the entire back side of the body.

You can roll your forearms on the lower leg, thigh, butt, or even on the back over the ribcage.

You can also apply elbow press around the hip, revisit the point of the boomerang etc.

To finish up iron the leg out with your forearms from the knee toward the heel and hip.

After you're done lift receiver's leg up and turn away from receiver only to swing your thai sitting to the other side and repeat the full sequence with the other leg and side.

Rec: Include this exercise in every session. It is so relaxing and comfy receivers like it a lot.

Bm: Thai sitting can be challenging at first. You can modify the sitting for yourself.

Sen Line: *Multiple*

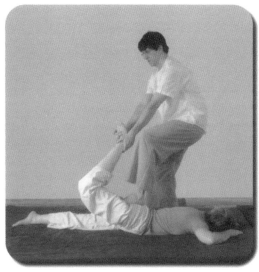

10.8 Leg stretch half locust

PP: Stand over one of receiver's leg in level with the knee facing away from her.

Pick up receiver's foot and bend the leg at the knee.

Prep: Lift up the bent leg and walk backward toward receiver's upper body and step out to the sides to have receiver's hip between your feet.

Exercise: When you reach the point of resistance place your same side foot over receiver's butt planting the ball of your foot below the Ischial Tuberosity.

Slowly raise the leg and press your foot in the same time.

This move requiers great sense of balance and sensitivity to perform the optimal stretch across the front of receiver's body.

Rec: Sometime receivers tend to hold their hip stiff and can't relax. Don't force this stretch if you feel strong holding in receiver.

Bm: Bend your knees. The pull should come from your knees, not from your back.

Eff: Great stretch for the front of the body and in the same time creates space in the gluteals and in the lower back.

Sen Line: *Sen Sahatsarangsi-Thawari, Sen Sumana*

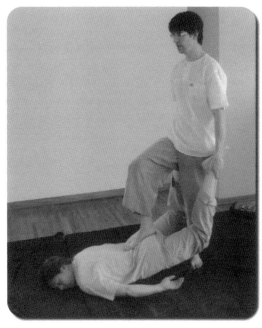

10.9 Wheelborrow

PP: Stand by receiver's feet.

Prep: Pick her legs up by the ankles.

Exercise: Let her legs relax and slowly walk toward receiver's hip between her legs.

Plant one of your foot between receiver's legs somewhere at the level of receiver's thigh and turn it to the side.

Pick up your other foot and place it on the sacrum.

Do not put pressure on it yet.

Slowly and slightly lean forward and transfer your body weight to your foot and rather pull the sacrum and lower back toward yourself to lengthen the spine.

Then move your foot from the sacrum and place it across the spine somewhere between the scapulas and transfer your body weight over it but this time with a forward direction to lengthen the spine toward receiver's head.

For the last of this sequence place your foot beside the spine on the same side and foot press the erector muscle group of the upper and mid back.

Then step back and repeat the sequence on the other side ith your other foot.

Rec: Make sure receiver is relaxed especially in the hips before you start the lengthening.

Bm: Let your arms hanging rather than pulling receiver's feet upward.

Make sure to turn your foot on the floor to the side to gain balance.

Eff: Stretches and lenghtens the body in the longitudinal direction.

Sen Line: *Multiple*

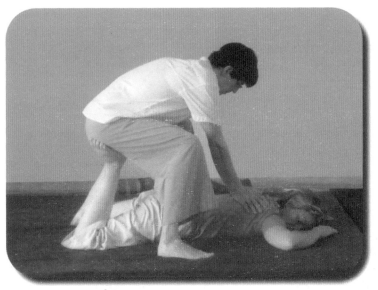

10.10 Palming, thumbing, palming back(E)

PP: Straddle over receiver's body in half kneeling or use receiver's feet as your stool.

Exercise: Palm the back alongside the spine between the iliac crest and the scapulas. You can alternate or double palm up and down several times.

Thumb the same area with both thumbs in the same time on the two sides of the spine up and down on the line between the spine and the erector muscle group, the line on the top of the erector muscle group and the line between the top of the iliac crest and the lower tip of the scapula.

Palm the entire area up and down to finish up.

Sen Line: *Multiple*

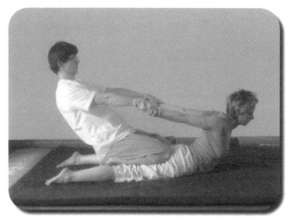

10.11 Cobra(E)

PP: Place your knees below receiver's Ischial Tuberosity and sit on your heels with your toes tucked under.

Choose to place your feet inside or outside of receiver's legs.

Prep: Start palming from the hip up on the back alongside the spine and this time continue the palming all the way up to the shoulders and to the arms down to the hands. It is a great transition move and makes your session and especially this exercise flowing.

Exercise: Grab receiver's wrist and ask her to grab on yours too.

Lift the arms up and open them to the side. Only after lean back to pull receiver up into the cobra. Release receiver back to the floor.

Repeat pulling up one more time ut this time rotate to the sides by adjusting the tension on the arms. Before releasing pull receiver up higher into the cobra again.

Ci: Lower back pain, surgery, injury.

Bm: Before pulling up receiver lift arms up and open them to the side.

If you miss this preparation you'll compress the lower back and cause more discomfort then stretch or release.

Eff: Stretches and lengthens the upper body.

The Cobra and the Wheelborrow(10.9) complement each other in a full body stretch.

Sen Line: *Sen Sumana, Sen Ittha-Pingkhala*

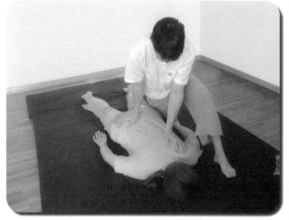

10.12 Back stretch(E)

PP: Straddle over receiver's body in half kneeling or halfkneel on the side.

Prep: Place your hands on the opposite "corners" of receiver's back, one over the scapula and the other above the opposite hip.

Exercise: Push your hands away from each other to create a stretch across the back.

Move your hands closer to each other and repeat the stretch and this time direct your press into the body. Move your hands apart again to the starting position and repeat the stretch. Repeat this sequence of stretches across the other "corners" of the back and along the spine.

Rec: Be carefull over the spine and direct your pressure to lengthen the back.

Eff: Relaxes and finishes the back position.

Sen Line: *Multiple*

Chapter 7
Sitting position

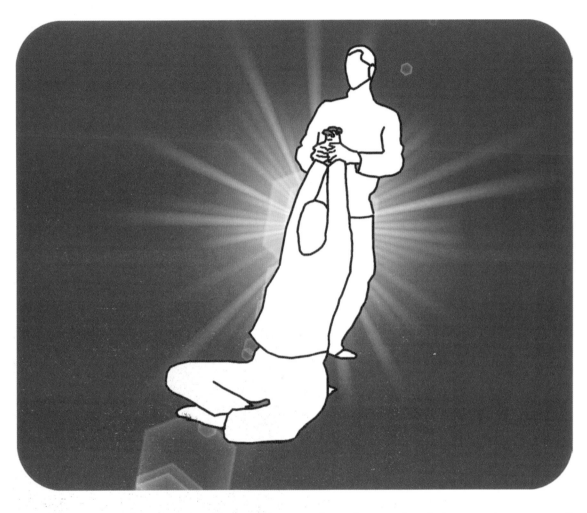

The Sitting position is the finale of our session. It is designed to bring receiver upward and back to the environment.

The main feature is the work with the shoulders and neck that the western life style affects the most. It is also recommended to extend the Back position, transitioning with bends and rotational exercises in the Sitting position. Make sure you have at least 10 minutes for this position to complete the session.

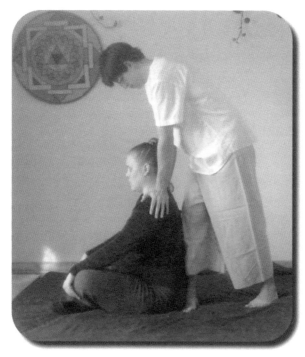

11.1 Palming thumbing palming shoulders(E)

PP: Stand behind receiver and plant one foot sideways right behind receiver to support her spine with your lower leg.

Exercise: Palm receiver's shoulder blades from the shoulder joint to the neck and back on both sides simultaneously.

When palming toward the neck hold your hands fingers resting on receiver's back and turn your hands to the front on the way back to the shoulders.

Follow the 1-2-3-2-1 pattern.

Rec: The pressure should be great on shoulders not superficial.

Bm: Transfer your upper body weight over your straight arms.

Sen Line: Sen Kalathari

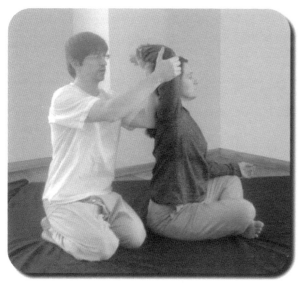

11.2.1 Water pump #1 (E)

PP: Kneel diagonally behind receiver toward the side that you're about to work with.

Prep: Lift receiver's arm up and bring her elbow to her ear and bend her arm.

Place your inside elbow between receiver's scapula and spine and grab receiver's wrist with the inside hand.

Place your outside hand on receiver's bent elbow from the front.

Exercise: Pull gently receiver's bent arm with both of your hands toward yourself and press your elbow against receiver's back.

Release and repeat it couple of times with changing the placing of your elbow around the scapula.

Rec: This exercise is a preparation for the next Water pump #2 Exercise 11.2.2. It can be used as assesment of the shoulder.

Sen Line: *Sen Kalathari*

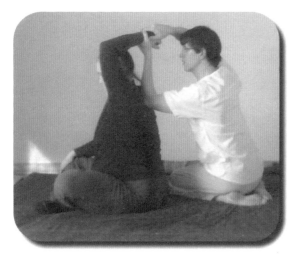

11.2.2 Water pump #2

PP: Kneel diagonally behind receiver toward the opposite side that you're about to work with.

Prep: Lift receiver's opposite arm up and bring her elbow to her ear and bend her arm.

Place your inside elbow between receiver's scapula and spine and grab receiver's wrist with both hands.

Exercise: Lean forward into receiver's back leading with your elbow and pull receiver's bent arm in the same time backward to create a full upper body stretch.

Release and repeat one more time.

Rec: The direciton of push with your elbow should be about 45 degrees toward the stretched side.

This is a serious stretch and receiver's with stiff or injured shoulder are not the best for it. For them use exercise 11.2.1 only.

Sen Line: *Sen Kalathari*

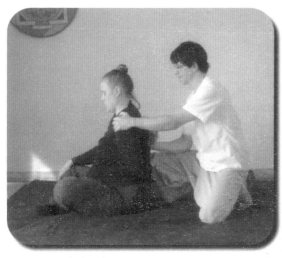

11.3 Palming thumbing palming around scapula(E)

PP: Kneeling behind receiver.

Prep: Pull receiver's hand back behind her back and place it on her back on the opposite side of her spine with palm out.

Place your knee in receiver's palm on her back and place your hand on the shoulder of her bent arm.

Exercise: Palm around the scapula with the edge of your inside hand and pull the shoulder back slightly to create counter force for the palming.

Palm down and up around the medial edge of scapula then change to thumbing.

Thumb the same area up and down several times.

Finish up with a round of palming.

Rec: Some receivers will not be able to get into the position. Do it with their arm on the same side.

Sen Line: *Sen Kalathari*

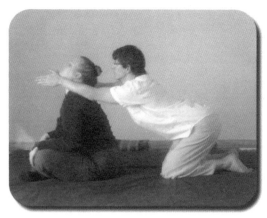

11.4 Neck stretch forward(E)

PP: Kneeling behind receiver.
Prep: Place both of your forearms on receiver's shoulders with your hands touching in the prayer position under her chin at the front of her neck.
Exercise: Press receiver's shoulders down with your forearms first and slowly move your hands upward lifting receivers chin up to create a stretch across the front of receiver's body then release.

Repeat this move 3 times.
Once with a turn to each sides and finally to the front again.
Rec: The key for this exercise is your lower back movement.
You need to flex your back similar to receiver's posture to be deep enough to create the stretch.
Bm: The stretch comes from your lower back and not so much from your arms.
Sen Line: *Sen Sumana, Sen Ittha-Pingkhala*

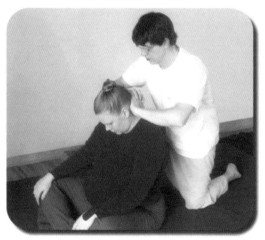

11.5 Neck palming and thumbing(E)

PP: Kneeling behind receiver.
Prep: Ask receiver to lower her head to expose the back of her neck.
Interlace your fingers over it.
Work with the lateral edges of the two big muscle ridges on each side of the spine.
Exercise: The palming turns into a nut-cracker motion as you press your palms together.
Palm the neck up and down many times.
The thumbing is like an ice-picker as you press your thumbs together.
Thumb also as long as you feel like it .
These are great exercises for the neck and everybody likes them.
Sen Line: *Sen Kalathari*

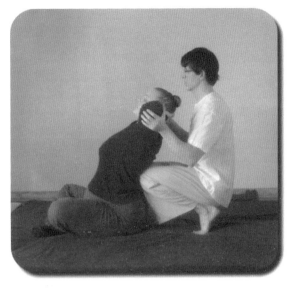

11.6 Springing(E)

PP: Kneeling behind receiver.
Prep: Ask receiver to interlace her fingers behind her neck.
Squat on your tip toes behind receiver and place your knees beside her spine on the middle back.
Hold her elbows from under in lower bird grasp.
Exercise: Slowly spring receiver back and forth supporting her back on your knees.
Adjust your knee position on receiver's back for every backward spring to change the effect and length of the stretch.
Repeat springing several times.
Rec: Hold receiver's elbow very lightly. The spring move should come from receiver and not from your arms. Use your arms for guiding.
Bm: This exercise requires great sense of balance as you're holding yourself on your tip toes.
Sen Line: *Sen Sumana*

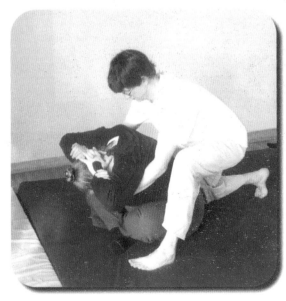

11.7 Assisted forward bend(E)

PP: Half kneeling behind receiver.
Prep: Ask her to interlace her hands on the back of her neck.
Swim your hands from the front into the triangle formed by receiver's upper and lower arms and grasp on her forearms.
Exercise: Take receiver into the forward bend then pull her back up.
Rec: If receiver is flexible enough hold her in forward bend position for a short while.
Sen Line: *Sen Sumana*

11.8 Spinal twist(E)

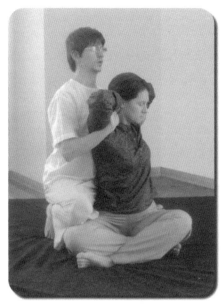

PP: Half kneeling behind receiver.

Prep: Ask her to interlace her hands on the back of her neck.

Swim your hands from the front into the triangle formed by receiver's upper and lower arms and grasp on her forearms.

In this position move toward receiver's side and place your front knee on receiver's thigh while lowering yourself on your heels.

Exercise: Pull receiver close to yourself pin her thigh with your knee and turn to the opposite direction into the spinal twist.

Release back to the front and move your knee on receiver's thigh closer to her body.

Repeat the spinal twist.

Release back to the front and move your knee on receiver's thigh closer to her body again.

Repeat the spinal twist for the last time.

After releasing receiver back to the front change side and repeat the spinal twist on the other side.

Bm: Pull receiver up and support her before start twisting.

Sen Line: *Sen Sumana*

11.9 Walking on the back(E)

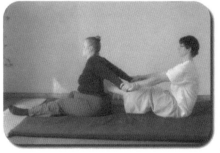

PP: Sitting behind receiver.

Prep: Bring her hands back and pull them behind.

Grab her wrists and ask her to grab your wrists as well.

Place your feet on receiver's back beside the spine.

Exercise: Walk up and down on receiver's back and hold her arms loose.

After covering the entire back with walking press both feet against receiver's back and gently pull her arms toward yourself by leaning backward.

Adjust your foot position on receiver's back and repeat the pull.

Repeat it many times.

Rec: This exercise creates a great stretch across receiver's front body especially across her chest.

The main feature although is the lengthening and straightening of the spine with the press of your feet.

Sen Line: *Sen Sumana, Sen Kalathari*

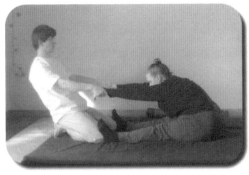

11.10 Front assisted forward bend with straight legs

PP: Move front of receiver and ask her to straight her legs out.

Sit on your heels with toes tucked under in kneeling.

Prep: Place your knees firmly on receiver's soles.

Come up into kneeling and ask for receiver's hands to hold them by the fingers.

Exercise: Slowly pull receiver into the forward bend by leaning back.

Repeat the forward bend couple of times.

After the last forward bend hold receiver's hands loose and shake them out.

Sen Line: *Sen Sumana*

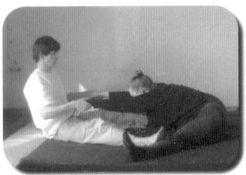

11.11.1 Front assisted forward bend with open legs

PP: Sitting front of receivers.

Prep: Ask receiver to open her legs as far as she can.

Place your feet on her lower legs inside below her knees.

Ask for receiver's hands and hold them by the fingers.

Exercise: Pull her into forward bend by leaning backward.

Repeat this forward bend couple of times.

Rec: Don't force the forward bend rather take receiver to the point of resistance and let her rest in the stretch.

Sen Line: *Multiple*

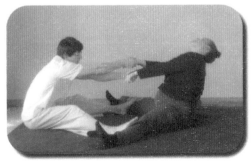

11.11.2 Front assisted spinning

PP: Sitting front of receiver.

Prep: Secure your sitting position by placing your feet against her legs below or above her knees with your heels on the floor.

Cross receiver's hands and hold them at the little finger side firmly.

Exercise: Move your upper body in a circle and simultaneously pull and push with your hands so receiver will follow your movement.

After several circles slow down and change direction to repeat the circles again.

Rec: Start the circular movement slowly and speed up just a bit as this exercise relaxing and loosening. It is not a rollercoaster ride!

Bm: The secret of this exercise is crossing receiver's arms not yours. Your arms need to be free while receiver's arms need to be fairly restricted to keep the control over her upper body.

Sen Line: *Sen Sahatsarangsi-Thawari*

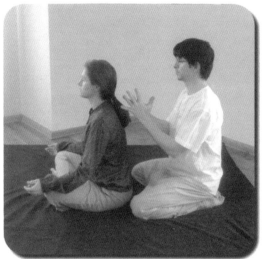

11.13 Percuss back(E)

PP: Kneeling behind receiver.

Prep: Put your hand in prayer position with fingers spread apart.

Exercise: Percuss receiver's entire upper back with loose fingers around the scapula and off of the spine.

The rhythm should be in sync with the flow of the session, slow but rhythmic, steady.

Your hands should make clapping noise when you do it right.

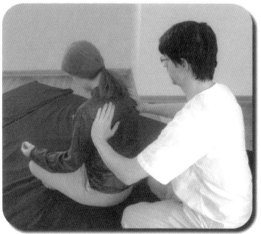

11.14 Sweep(E)

PP: Kneeling behind receiver.

Prep: Place your hands on her spine just below the neck.

Exercise: Sweep your hands with fingers apart on the shoulder blades once, across the scapulas once, across the mid back once and move back up across the scapulas and finish with a sweep across the the shoulder blades.

Rec: I like to use the last line fom the Om Namo Sivago mantra with the sweeps:

NA-A, NA-WA, ROKHA, PAYATI, VINA SANTI

PART III
SEN LINE ANATOMY

Sen Line Anatomy

Most of fellow Thai massage practitioners would frown their eyebrows upon reading the title above so I explain it before I roll out the concept of correspondence between Prana or Qi energy flow and anatomy, which I think makes sense. I see it as the beauty of nature and the human design in it reflecting throughout different cultures and believe systems. I also think it is a start of unifying east and west, modern and ancient within the field of healing. In practice, it gives Thai massage practitioners the profound understanding of the 3 dimensional physical nature of the body of energy, and they can identify its sections and their connections under their hands, for more efficient work and better outcome. So instead of keep dividing and reducing our healing art into new styles or modalities I prefer to unify it with other great science and arts.

The scope of this book and this part of it are limited to show the resemblance between the theories of two seemingly different healing practices the Thai Energy Lines and the Anatomy Trains myofascial meridians. Therefore the information collected and discussed here will not fully present them, rather meant to give better insight about the spectrum of Thai massage.

The Energy Line theory - The Energy

There are two major cultures from the past the Chinese and the Indian that concluded the same principal of life which is the vital force or Qi in Chinese and Prana in Sanskrit, both means breath. Interestingly the first written chinese text is from 479 B.C. during the time of the Yellow Emperor which is about the time of Buddha in India.
The chinese connecting this vital force or energy flow to the creation of the universe and everything in it as follows:

„...Universe produces Qi, Qi has bounds. The clear, yang [qi] was ethereal and so formed heaven. The heavy, turbid [qi] was congealed and impeded and so formed earth. The conjunction of the clear, yang [qi] was fluid and easy. The conjunction of the heavy, turbid [qi] was strained and difficult. So heaven was formed first and earth was made fast later. The pervading essence (xi-jing) of heaven and earth becomes yin and yang. The concentrated (zhuan) essences of yin and yang become the four seasons. The dispersed (san) essences of the four seasons become the myriad creatures. The hot qi of yang in accumulating produces fire. The essence (jing) of the fire-qi becomes the sun. The cold qi of yin in accumulating produces water. The essence of the water-qi becomes the moon. The essences produced by coitus (yin) of the sun and moon become the stars and celestial markpoints (chen, planets)."

Theories of traditional Chinese medicine assert that the body has natural patterns of qi that circulate in channels called meridians in English. Symptoms of various illnesses are often believed to be the product of disrupted, blocked, or unbalanced qi movement (interrupted flow) through the body's meridians, as well as deficiencies or imbalances of qi (homeostatic imbalance) in the various Zang Fu organs. Traditional Chinese medicine often seeks to relieve these imbalances by adjusting the circulation of qi (metabolic energy flow) in the body using a variety of therapeutic techniques. Some of these techniques include herbal medicines, special diets, physical training regimens (qigong, tai chi chuan, and other martial arts training), moxibustion, massage to clear blockages, and acupuncture, which uses small diameter metal needles inserted into the skin and underlying tissues to reroute or balance qi.

On the other hand the Indian Prana is one of the five organs of vitality or sensation, Prana is the breath, the others are speech, sight, hearing, and thought (nose, mouth, eyes, ears and mind). Its most subtle material form is the breath.
In Vedantic philosophy, it is the notion of a vital, life-sustaining force of living beings. Prana is a central concept in Ayurveda and Yoga where it is believed to flow through a network of fine subtle channels called nadis.
Prana was first expounded in the Upanishads, where it is part of the worldly, physical realm, sustaining the body and the mother of thought and thus also of the mind. Prana suffuses all living forms but is not itself the Atman or individual soul. In the Ayurveda, the sun and sunshine are held to be a source of Prana.
Pranayama is the practice in which the control of prana is achieved (initially) from the control of one's breathing. According to Yogic philosophy the breath, or air, is merely a gateway to the world of prana and its manifestation in the body. In yoga, pranayama techniques are used to control the movement of these vital energies within the body, which is said to lead to an increase in vitality in the practitioner.

The Energy Line theory - The Lines

The Indian Energy Line theory is more interesting to us, because Thai massage have borrowed its 10 Energy Lines from the Yoga tradition. The Chinese energy lines or Chinese Meridians are representing the connection between the inside of the body - the internal organs - and the outside. It is clear that they have similar source but the application and routing is different from the Thai or the Indian Energy Lines. (If you interested to find correspondence with Chinese meridians take a look at Richard Gold's Thai massage book).

according to the yoga tradition there are 72000 energy lines!

If we use our western knowledge and perception it sounds overwhelming, way too many to deal with or even draw them with a computer. So there has to be some other way to sort them out. The theory is laid out in one of my favorite book the Brightness of the East from Kaczvinszky as follows:

By observing the Indian energy system of the body we find 7 Chakras along the spine, and really along the upper body. The Chakras located (from bottom to top) at the base of the spine, the lower belly, below the navel, at the level of the heart, at the throat, in the middle of the forehead between the eyebrows and on the top of the head.
Connecting each neighboring Chakras there is a manifestation responsible for certain characteristics of the person.
These are:
the *Stature* between the 1st and 2nd Chakras,
the *Abilities* between the 2nd and 3rd Chakras,
the *Thinking* skill between the 3rd and 4th Chakra,
the *Character* between the 4th and 5th Chakras,
the *Buddhi* between the 5th and 6th Chakras and,
the *Individual psyche* between the 6th and 7th Chakras.

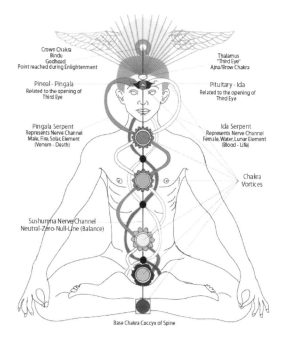

All of these 6 manifestations contain all the 6 manifestations. That makes 36 variations all together. The Crown Chakra has a special property, as some of the translations are pointing to it, so as the symbol of the lotus flower or the wheel. It is really means infinite that Indians has translated as 1000. It is now 36000 variations. Because every Chakra has left and right sides (Ida and Pingala), the number of possible characteristics of these manifestations are twice as much.
So the formula of the 72000 Energy Lines is this:

$$6 \times 6 \times 1000 \times 2 = 72000$$

Illustration 9. The Chakras(Reproduced with kind permission from Gary Osborn)

The whole Chakra system is out of the scope of this book but the basics are crucial to understand the theory of the Energy Lines.

In the Indian theory of Energy really the Chakra system is the main installment.
There are three main channels of prana along the Chakra system are Ida, Pingala and Sushumna. Ida relates to the left side of the body, terminating at the left nostril. Ida symbolizes the moon, the female power and the reception. Pingala means the right side of the body, the sun, the male power and penetration, terminating at the right nostril.

Here is the point where Thai massage has direct connection to Yoga tradition as the first 3 Energy Lines in Thai massage are Sen Sumana, Sen Ittha, Sen Pingkhala. These are the very same names as in the Yoga tradition. The connection to India and to the Yoga tradition is obvious as we discussed it earlier in the History of Thai Massage in Part I., but these names and their description are identical while the rest of the history calls for further research.

Thai massage did extend the Chakra system further, to include all parts of the body. I was thaught that Thais selected their energy Lines from the original 72000 Indian nadis but most likely it happened different way. The 3 main Energy Lines Ida, Pingala and Sushumna got extended to the arms and the legs and became Sen Ittha, Sen Pingkhala, and Sen Sumana, then several new sets of Energy Lines have been introduced and mapped out. The first complete map of the Sib Sen was published by Asokananda and Chow Kam Thye .

These are the *Sib Sen* (Ten Lines):
Sen Sumana
Sen Ittha – Sen Pingkhala
Sen Kalathari
Sen Sahatsarangsi - Sen Thawari
Sen Lawusang - Sen Ulangka
Sen Nanthakravat - Sen Khitchanna

Other part of Indian theory is also handy in the practice of Thai massage. It is the theory of the 5 Koshas and the Atman. Again I don't attempt to give it in whole, but the stimulation of the Energy Flow can be confusing without it. We are really focusing on the first two Koshas which are the Physical body or Annamaya kosha and the Energy body or Pranamaya kosha. Massaging and stretching the body we are in direct contact with the Physical body, and our attention goes straight to the Energy body (Pranamaya kosha). These sheaths or layers are in constant connection and relation to each other so easy to understand that physical symptoms can affect the deeper layers, and deeper layers can affect the outer layer of the body which is the case in Thai massage. So in Thai massage we really sensing the energy flow and its manifestations in the physical body and making interventions through the physical structures.

The 5 koshas by the Yoga tradition:

Kosha means sheath, like the lampshades covering the light. Maya means appearance, as if something appears to be one way, but is really another. Advaita Vedanta suggests that you imagine a dark night in which you think you see a man, only to find that it was an old fence post that was hard to see at first; that is maya.
The Yoga path of Self-realization is one of progressively moving inward, through each of those bodies, so as to experience the purity at the eternal center of consciousness, while at the same time allowing that purity to animate through our individuality.
The five levels or koshas:

Physical - Annamaya kosha
This is the sheath of the physical self, named from the fact that it is nourished by food. Living through this layer man identifies himself with a mass of skin, flesh, fat, bones, and filth, while the man of discrimination knows his own self, the only reality that there is, as distinct from the body.

Energy - Pranamaya kosha
Pranamaya means composed of prana, the vital principle, the force that vitalizes and holds together the body and the mind. It pervades the whole organism, its physical manifestation is the breath. As long as this vital principle exists in the organisms, life continues. Coupled with the five organs of action it forms the vital sheath.

Mental - Manamaya kosha
Manomaya means composed of manas or mind. The mind (manas) along with the five sensory organs is said to constitute the manomaya kosa. The manomaya kohsa, or "mind-sheath" is said more truly to approximate to personhood than annamaya kosha and pranamaya kosha. It is the cause of diversity, of I and mine.

Wisdom - Vijnanamaya kosha
Vijnanamaya means composed of intellect, the faculty which discriminates, determines or wills. It is the combination of intellect and the five sense organs. It is the sheath composed of more intellection, associated with the organs of perception.

Bliss - Anandamaya kosha
Anandamaya means composed of ananda, or bliss. In the Upanishads the sheath is known also as the causal body. In deep sleep, when the mind and senses cease functioning, it still stands

between the finite world and the self. Anandamaya, or that which is composed of Supreme bliss, is regarded as the innermost of all. The bliss sheath normally has its fullest play during deep sleep: while in the dreaming and wakeful states, it has only a partial manifestation.

Self - Atman
Atman is the Self, the eternal center of consciousness, which was never born and never dies. In the metaphor of the lamp and the lampshades, Atman is the light itself, though to even describe it as that is incomplete and incorrect. The deepest light shines through the koshas, and takes on their colorings.
It means that each of the sheaths or koshas is only an appearance. In truth, all of the levels, layers, koshas, or sheaths of our reality is only appearance, or maya (while also very real in the sense of dealing with the external world), and that underneath all of those appearances, we are pure, divine, eternal consciousness, or whatever name you prefer to call it.

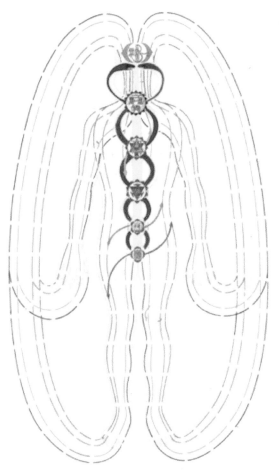

Also important part of the Indian tradition is the Aura which is the glowing rainbow colored bubble around every "living" thing. In Thai massage we don't use any manipulation aimed to the aura, but it can be a subject of study to show what kind of changes happen during or after a Thai massage session. I know it would be very interesting as I heard that Rolfing creates a nice blue healing aura, shared by therapist and client. I've found this great aura picture, the first that really shows the connectedness of the arms and legs to the Aura as a whole.

Illustration 10. Lines of energy and the Chakras(from public domain)

The myofascial meridians

After all these remote knowledge about ourselves, there are hypothetical theories that suggest qi or prana could be transmitted through the fascia independent of any neurological activity.

Also more recent investigations point to the mechano-transduction ability of the connective tissue, in other words a domino effect caused by the specific twisting and knotting of the fabric of the body . The connections with electric conductivity were studied in the United States in the late 19th Century, and are currently the subject of more active research.

What is this really means?
How the fascia, the connective tissue comes into the picture?

It happened to me when I first looked at Thomas Myers' book the Anatomy Trains. Its cover picture looked like the Thai Sen Lines laid over Albinus' anatomical figure which I knew weren't the case. Or was it? So I purchased the book and started to learn about fascia and anatomy, tensegrity, double bag theory, etc.

To understand the optical illusion that happened to me I introduce the connective tissue and inviting you to reeducate yourself about the bone-muscle or the single muscle concept that presented in standard anatomical atlases and descriptions.
Please note that this part of the book presents a point of view that geared toward the attempt to unite knowledge about ourselves and is by no means the complete story of fascia or the living force or energy theory.

In medias res, I skip the whole evolution theory and the Gods or higher powers of creation and I jump right into the cell specialization of the human body. After the original ovum goes through the multiplication of stem cells, differentiation takes place. It creates four basic types of cells that then combined into tissues, organs, organisms and societies. These are the epithelial, muscle, nerve and connective tissue cells. Each of these cells have different abilities to contract, secrate, conduct. The connective tissue cells are lousy at contraction, not very good at condution but they very good secrating. They so good at it that they produce a variety of prodcucts into the intercellular space that contribute to our bones, cartliage, ligamnets, tendons and more.

According to Tom Myers:

„... In other words, it is these cells which create the surroundings for all the others, building the strong, pliable 'stuff' which holds us together, forming the shared and communicative environment for all our cells, shaping us and allowing us directed movement..."

At this point I would bring up the previously introduced Energy body or Pranamaya kosha:

Pranamaya means composed of prana, the vital principle, the force that vitalizes and holds together the body and the mind. It pervades the whole organism; its physical manifestation is the breath. As long as this vital principle exists in the organisms, life continues. Coupled with the five organs of action it forms the vital sheath.

I wasn't expected this much resemblance but now looks like there are some shared views about the function of these very different systems.

If we change the microscope to x-ray vision and looking at the human body as a whole we can find 3 holistic networks. The first is the neural net, the sum ammount of nerves of the body. The second is the fluid net, the vascular system, starting with the heart and the major arteries and veins all the way down to the capillaries. The third is the fibrous network - made up by the connective tissue - with all the particles of it such as collagen, elastin, reticulin and others. I think Tom Myers description of the fibrous net worth to read:

„The bones, cartliage, tendons, and ligaments would be thick leathery fiber, so that the area around each joint would be especially well-represented. Each muscle would be sheathed with it, and infused with a cotton-candy net surrounding each muscle cell and bundle of cells. The face would be less dens, as would the more spongy organs. Though even these would be surrounded by one or two denser, tough bags. Although it arranges itself in folded planes, we emphasize once again that no part of this net would be distinct or separated from the net as a whole; each of these bags, strings, sheets, and leathery networks is linked to each other, top to toe. The center of this network would be our mechanical center of gravity, located in the middle of the lower belly in the standing body.
The bald statement is that, like the neural and vascular web so permeates the body as to be part of the immediate environment of every cell. Without its support, the brain would be runny custard, the liver would spread through the abdominal cavity, and we would end up as a puddle at our own feet. Only in the open lumens of the respiratory and digestive tracts is the binding, strengthening, connecting, and separating web of fascia absent. Even in the circulatory tubes, filled with flowing blood, itself a connective tissue, the potential exists for fiber to form at any

moment we need a clot.

We could not extract a cubic centimeter, let alone Shylock's pound of flesh, without encountering this meshwork of collagen. With any touch more than feathery light, we contact the tone of this web, registering it wheter we are conscious of it or not, and affecting it, whatever our intention."

After a short digestion of the information above with our scalpel sharp visualization, a whole bunch of knowledge of anatomy and a handful of rules by Tom Myers we can isolate the myofascial meridians (longitudinal connective tissue links) in the context of the whole body.

These are:

The Superficial Front Line (SFL),

The Superficial Back Line (SBL),

The Lateral Line (LL),

The Spiral Line (SL),

The Arm Lines (SFAL, DFAL, SBAL, DBAL),

The Functional Lines (FFL,BFL),

The Deep Front Line (DFL).

I strongly emphasize that this is only possible by removing and dissolving hundreds of millions of other connections within the connective tissue and the body, therefore it is just one set of possible meridians – playing main role in posture - and these never exist or function by themselves alone in the living body.

Oh, just one more thing: to be in the gravitational electromagnetic field with the earth ithat is what organizes the living structures like the human body…

The 10 Energy Lines
(Sib Sen)

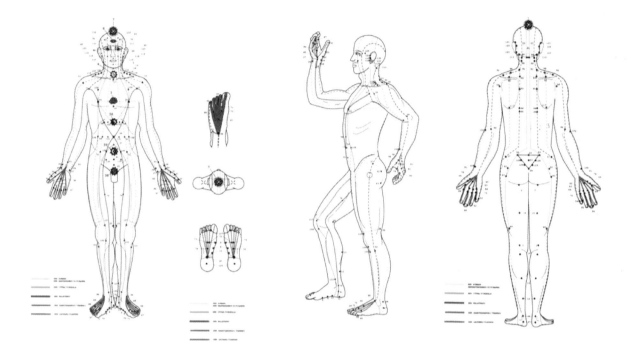

Illustration 11. The Ten Sen Lines by Asokananda(Reproduced with kind permission from Andrea Baglioni)

The rest of this part of the book demonstrates each Sen Lines and the corresponding longitudinal myofascial units. First is the presentation of the Sen Energy Lines with its descrpitions, according to Andrea Baglioni who has redrawn them from Asokananda's heritage. Then I show the corresponding longitudinal myofascial unit with proper anatomical description with plate references for Frank H. Netter's ATLAS OF HUMAN ANATOMY, published by CIBA-Geigy, although you can follow with any good anatomy atlas. Then you'll find the specific exercises for each Sen Line.

The anatomical descriptions of these meridians and the referenced pictures show great detail of them. Muscle names and other anatomical terms are used like zip codes of the body to direct our attention to specific part or section of the fascial net.

Sen Sumana

Illustration 12. Sen Sumana(Reproduced with kind permission from Andrea Baglioni)

Indications, therapy

Asthma, bronchitis, chest pain, heart disease, spasm of the diaphragm, nausea, cold, cough, throat problems, diseases of digestive system, abdominal pain, back pain

Tracing

Sen Sumana runs from the side of the big toe with one branch arching off after the ball of the foot running right below the bony structure of the foot, the other branch runs straight to the heel where they joining again. It continues around the inside of the heel and onto the Achilles tendon (3rd inside line on the calf) and then between the split muscle after the Achilles tendon to the centre of the back of the knee.

Here the line splits into two, with one branch continuing above the hamstring on the inside of the leg to the pubic bone, the other branch running straight from the back of the knee to the buttock bone and from there to the coccyx.

From the pubic bone the line runs in the centre of the body through the centre of the sternum and the throat to the centre of the face and the centre of the forehead, covering all the 6 major chakras on the way then moving into the Crown Chakra in the centre of the top of the head.

On heart level the line branches out across the chest and crossing the nipples and follows the edge of the armpit towards the inside of the arms and inside the bone towards the side of the little finger. Above the collar bone the line branches out across the shoulders towards the inside of the arms and inside the bone towards the side of the thumbs.

From the coccyx the line runs in the centre of the sacrum on the spine towards the head where it moves into the Crown Chakra.

The arm line towards the little fingers Sen Sumana shares with Sen Ittha-Pingkhala, while the arm line towards the thumbs Sen Sumana shares with Sen Sahatsarangsi-Thawari.

Exercises - Sen Sumana
Foot massage
1.1, 1.3, 1.12 medial arch
Lines on the leg
Palming and thumbing 3rd inside line on the legs in supine position
2.2, 2.3, 2.4
Single leg exercises
3.4, 3.6, 3.13, 3.14, 3.15, 3.17, 3.18, 3.20, 3.21, 3.24, 3.25
Double leg exercises
4.1, 4.2, 4.3, 4.4, 4.5, 4.9, 4.10, 4.11,
Front upper body
6.2,
Side position
9.2, 9.22.1, 9.22.2
Back position
10.3, 10.4, 10.8, 10.11
Sitting position
11.4, 11.6, 11.7, 11.8, 11.9, 11.10

The Deep Front Line - DFL

Before going into details of this myofascial meridian, I need to say that the correspondance between the Sen Sumana and the DFL is stunning. It is a bit surprising to me because this is the deepest in the body and maybe the most diverse fascially connected of all the myofascial meridians. Also Sen Sumana is the main Sen Line of all and seeing, sensing this Energy Line requires special skills that masters of the past obviously possessed.

Looking at the The Deep Front Line - also called the core or core line - from the bottom to the top, it starts with the long toe flexors, the Flexor digitorum longus, the Flexor hallucis longus and the Tibialis posterior muscle (Netter Plate 502). All three of them attach at the plantar surface of the foot. These tendons then emerge from the bottom of the foot - what you can see in Sen Sumana has the same pathway as the flexor hallucis longus from the big toe – and form the muscles of the deep posterior compartment of the lower leg. The muscles then attach to the tibia, fibula and interosseous membrane between them (Netter Plate 487).

From here the fascial connection leads us up to the back side of the Popletius muscle. The muscle fibers of the Popletius are across but the fascial fibers on the back side of it are connecting right into the knee capsule (Netter Plate 480). Just for expanding our understanding of the fascial net, the neurovascular bundle also part of this fascial continuum behind the knee joint capsule. The DFL links up through the Adductor hiatus to the adductor group. If you look at Sen Sumana you'll see clearly the 3rd inside line following the Gracilis muscle which is the midline of the whole adductor group. But what about the branch line on the middle of the back of the leg? Is that associated with the hamstrings? It make sense by directionally but depth wise the hamstrings are too superficial. I think it must be the attachments of the adductors "around" the Linea aspera (Netter Plate 465).

From the top of the legs the DFL braches out into different tracks (Netter Plate 466). One track is following the Iliacus and runs over the iliac crest to the QL to attach to the Diaphragm and the spine which is important to us. The second track goes through Pectinius muscle and the Lacunar ligament to attach to the Psoas minor which eventually weave in with the Diaphragm and the Anterior longitudinal ligament. The 3rd track is the (an express track by AT terms) Psoas major bridging over the hip joint and hangs on the lumbar spine. These are the bigger muscles of the hip but if we think of Sen Sumana, it includes the Chakras from the bottom of the spine which we know, all are 3 dimentional. The lower 3 Chakras are the Root Chakra, the Sex Chakra and the center of gravity in the 2nd Chakra and the Solar plexus in the 3rd.

The Root Chakra easilly can be seen corresponding with the pelvic floor - which is also in relation to all other domes of the body, like the arches of the foot, the Diaphragm, the floor and the roof of the mouth etc- and part of the DFL.

The Sex Chakra symbolizes the organs of the reproduction system which are the content of the abdominal cavity with the mesentery and the internal organs. The interesting is that the posterior and inferior walls of this cavity forms the DFL that we discussed above.

The Solar plexus the 3rd Chakra located at the junction of the Psoas and the Diaphragm which is just front of the Thoraco-Lumbar hinge of the spine (Netter Plate 246).

 If you look at the indication of Sen Sumana we can find spasm of the diaphragm, nausea, diseases of digestive system, abdominal pain, back pain. Make sense?

Continue up with the 2 domes of the Diaphragm we can see several fascial connections like the one is to the mediastium (to the heart, the ribcage, through the lungs, etc. (Netter Plate 200)), then straight up to the throat then to the floor of the mouth with muscles like the Digastric, Mylohyoid, Geniohyoid and the tounge itself. These fascial connections lead us to the 4th Chakra which is the Heart Chakra, then to the Fifth which is the Throat Chakra.

Now, we know that the top point of Sen Sumana is in the Crown Chakra on the top of the head, but we won't find a single muscle connecting from the neck to up there on the front of the face, neither on the middle of the back of the head. What we actually have is a combinations of fascial connections (Netter Plate 24,25) on either side of the head through the jaw muscles or the pterygoids and fascia across the head and mechanical connections through the skull and of course through the brain - which is in touch with the 6th Chakra the Third Eye- and its multiple layers of fascia around it.

Sen Ittha (left side of the body), Sen Pingkhala (right side of the body)

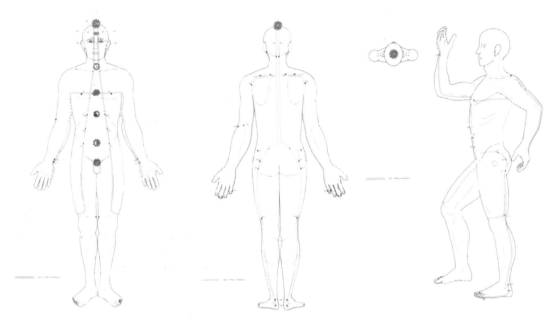

Illustration 13. Sen Ittha-Pingkhala(Reproduced with kind permission from Andrea Baglioni)

Indications, therapy

Headache, stiff neck, shoulder pain, common cold, cough, nasal obstruction, sore throat, sore eyes, chill and fever, abdominal pain, intestinal diseases, back pain, diseases of the urinary track, dizziness, all internal organs

Additional indication to Sen Pingkhala: Diseases of liver and the gall bladder

Tracing

Sen-Ittha-Pingkhala run from the side of the little toe around the outside of the heel towards the calf on the outside of the lower leg between the Achilles tendon and the calf bone, close to the calf bone (3rd outside line). From there they move across the side of the knee towards the outside of the thigh running between the hamstring and the bone towards the buttocks. There they turn in a big boomerang towards the highest tip of the hip bone.

Right above the knees the lines split up and the branches move in a gentle arch onto the inside of the leg forming the 1st inside line on the thigh. The lines continue across the groin towards the abdomen, where they cover the abdomen points, one thumb distant from the navel. They then continue in the form of a wide funnel towards the side of the sternum, the throat and the face, run across the tear ducts and then enter the 6th Chakra

124

at the sides of the Chakra, then they energetically link up with Sen Sumana and reach up to the 7th Chakra on the top of the head. On heart level the lines branch out across the chest and across the nipples and around the edge of the armpits towards the inside of the arms and inside the bone towards the side of the little lingers.
The arm line towards the inside of the little fingers Sen Ittha-Pingkhala share with Sen Sumana.

Before the lines turn into the boomerang on the side of the body a branch splits off moving across the buttocks to the top of the sacrum and from there forming the 1st backlines right next to the spine. The lines continue towards the head running right next to the spine and next to the neck vertebrae towards the base of the skull and onto the head, where the lines move into the 7th Chakra.
Right above the shoulder blades the lines branch out towards the outside of the arms and towards the outside the little fingers.

Exercises - Sen Ittha-Pingkhala
Lines of the leg
Thumbing and palming the 1st inside line on the thigh
1.12 lateral side, 3.22, 3.23
Front upper body
5.3, 6.2, 6.3,7.1, 7.2, 7.3 additional technique,7.4,8.1
Side Position
9.4.1, 9.4.2, Palming and thumbing the 3rd outside line of the leg
9.5, 9.6, 9.7, 9.8, 9.9, 9.10, 9.11,9.19, 9.20 additional technique, 9.21
Back position
10.7, 10.1010.11
Sitting position
11.1, 11.4 to the sides,

The Lateral Line - LL

As you can see I left the Chakras on the Ittha Pingkhala lines chart. My intention whit it is to spotlight the hidden nature of these lines which is to create and maintain balance to open up Sen Sumana. When Ittha and Pingkhala are unbalanced Sumana will not function fully. Interestingly the Lateral Line has similar balancing function, posturally connect and balance the the front and back, bilaterally balance the left and right. They work like laces on the side of the body. Also, if we look deeper into the body we'll find matching pathways.

The starting point of the Lateral Line at the foot are the 1st and 5th metatarsal bases. If we look at Sen Ittha and Pingkhala only the 5th metatarsal involved with the outside of the foot. The Fibularis brevis and longus are going posterior and lateral to the lateral malleolus and connect from here up the the posterior side of the fibular head (Netter Plate 490). These muscles supporting the medial longitudinal arch of the foot amongs their other functions. From the Fibula the LL swithes through the anterior ligament of the head of the fibula to the Illiotibial band and leads us up to the Iliac crest, ASIS, PSIS employing Tensor fascia latae, Gulteus maximus and medius forming a "Y" shape.

Sen Ittha-Pingkhala clearly takes the space between Biceps femoris and Vastus lateralis (Netter Plate 464) which is one of my favorite formation in the human body, a septum between two different group of myofascial units. We will see more and more that Sen lines running along these septums.

Moving upward toward the glutes we bump into the boomerang of Ittha-Pingkhala. We notice in practice that each receiver has different sensations during the elbow work over these boomerang points. Soon it turns out that these points are located over not only the glutes but over the deep lateral rotators. Namely Qatratus femoris at Point 1, Periformis at Point 2 and Gluteus medius-minimus at Point 3. (Netter Plate 465). Unfortunatley other than the Gluteus medius-minimus these myofascial units don't fit into the Anatomy Trains theory as they do not have direct linear fascial continuity to the rest of the LL. But energetically and balance and posture wise they very important; supporting the pelvic floor, giving suspention to the hip, contributing to high-low and tilted hip patterns, etc.

From here LL fascially connects to both the External and Internal obliques. These muscles are crossing over each other forming an "X" shape linking up to the ribs where the fascial connections continue to the rib bones and the Intercoastals (Netter Plate 183).

Looking at this Netter plate I have a feeling about the significance of the LL and Sen Ittha-Pingkhla in breathing. The Scalene muscles will come up later but they fit right into the picture. At this level Ittha-Pingkhala run on the front of the body – from the inside of the knees – and form the 6 points of the abdomen. These points positioned over the lateral edge of the Rectus abdominis where the obliques weave into the rectus sheath (Netter Plate 233).

Before we continue up on the ribs we can find fascial connections to the Gall bladder at the Obliques but it isn't part of the LL, though if you look at the indications of Ittha-Pingkhala on the previous page you'll see mentioning the Gall bladder. Hm.
Jumping up to the top of the ribcage the LL concludes in the Scalene muscles that support the ribcage off of the transverse processes of the neck. The final part of the LL is the "X" combined by the SCM and the Splenius attaches at the Mastoid process and the Occiput.

Sen Ittha-Pingkhala follows the front of the body and it is important to us at this point that The Sen Energy Lines are not presented on the side of the torso. Instead Sen Ittha-Pingkhala connect up paralell to Sen Sumana all the way to the top of the head.
The feature of Sen Ittha-Pingkhala though make sense as the 2nd lines of the back. That is the pathway of the deepest expression of the LL, the tiny Intertransversarii muscles that run from transverse process to transvers process in the spine. They are involved in swimming and walking movments respectively.

Sen Kalathari

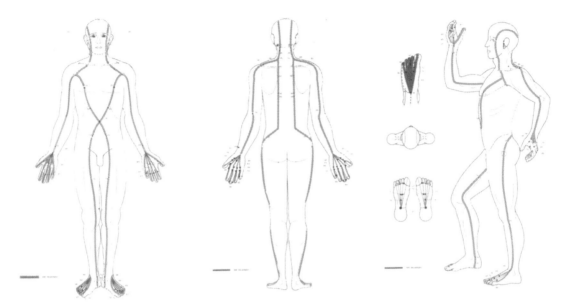

Illustration 14. Sen Kalathari(Reproduced with kind permission from Andrea Baglioni)

Indications, therapy
Diseases of digestive system indigestion, hernia, paralysis of arms and legs, knee pain, jaundice, whooping cough, arthritis of the fingers, chest pain, shock, rheumatic heart disease and cardiac arrhythmia, sinusitis, pain in arms and legs, angina pectoris, epilepsy, schizophrenia, hysteria, various psychic diseases and mental disorders.

Tracing
Sen Kalathari runs from the centre of the sole of the foot right front of the heel in fan form towards all the toes then folding over to the dorsum of the foot at the toes, running in fan form to the indentation between the foot and the leg in the centre of the dorsum of the foot. From the point right before the heel in the centre of the sole of the foot the lines run to the inside of the leg forming the 2nd inside lines on the legs. They continue up across the centre of the groin towards the navel, where an energy criss-cross takes place. From the navel they run across the nipples and the centre of the front of the shoulder onto the inside of the arms, forming the 2nd or central arm line below the bicep muscle on the upper arm and in the centre of the lower arm. At the wrist the line forms a fan towards all the fingers.

At the centre of the front of the shoulder a branch of the line moves up along the side of the throat towards the outer edge of the eye socket, from where it continues in a half circle around the side of the head towards the base of the skull and an indentation just below the base of the skull.

From the indentation between the foot and the leg in the centre of the dorsum of the foot the lines run up the legs as the 2nd outside lines of the leg just above the calf bone on the calf and in the center of the thigh. It then runs across the buttocks crossing the boomerang at the third boomerang point of the hip bone moving towards the back forming the 2nd back line on the muscular ridge between the spine and the shoulder blade and continues along the back side of the neck towards the indentation below the base of the skull.

In the soft area above the shoulders the lines branch towards the outside of the arms forming the 2nd outside lines in the centre of the outside of the arms. At the wrist the line forms a fan towards all the fingers.

Exercises
Foot massage
1.4, 1.5, 1.7, 1.8, 1.9, 1.10
Lines on the leg
Palming and thumbing 2nd inside and outside lines on the legs in supine position
2.8
Single leg exercises
3.2, 3.5, 3.8v, 3.10, 3.12, 3.21
Double leg exercises
4.6, 4.8
Front upper body
5.1, 5.2, 6.4, 7.1, 7.2, 7.3, 7.5-7.11, 8.1,
Side position
9.8-9.21
Back position
10.1, 10.2, 10.10
Sitting position
11.1, 11.2.2, 11.3, 11.5, 11.9

Superficial Back Line, Front Functional Line - SBL, FFL

Sen Kalathari is one of the most mysterious line of all Sen lines. One of its main property is the connectedness to the vascular system as you can see heart disease, and cardiac arrhythmia amongs the indications. If you look at the tracing of the line you'll see Sen Kalathari is the 2nd Energy line everywhere and all the blood stops are on the 2nd line. Also Sen Kalathari has known as a gateway between the 2nd Kosah the Energy body and the 3rd Kosah of the mind.

The tracing of Sen Kalathari gave me the biggest challenge finding corresponding myofascial meridian. And that was the trap I set up for myself because there is no one myofascial meridian that would cover this much teritory with the characteristics of crossing the body and still would make sense. I've ended up recruiting three meridians of the Anatomy Trains to make it work then I refined the result and settled with two sets of myofascial meridians. Let's see the details of front, back and crossing.

Sen Kalathari covers both plantar, palmar and dorsal sides of the feet and the hands. That already makes me think of back and front balance and antagonism. If we follow the flexors and extensors from the feet we can identify two major myofascial meridians the Superficial Front Line and the Superficial Back Line. From the tip of the toes the Extensor digitorum and hallucis longus lead us up to the anterior and lateral side of the lower leg. These muscles are part of the Superficial Front Line as an alternate track - the main aspect of the SFL comprised of the Tibialis anterior, the knee cap and the Rectus femoris will present the next sets of Sen lines- to the head of the Fibula and into the anterior edge of the Iliotibial band (Netter Plate 490, 464).

From the sides of the hips Sen Kalathari turn to the back crossing the 3rd boomerang point and form the 2nd back lines on the top of the erector group and lead us up all the way to the head (Netter Plate 161), where the lines folding over it and joining with the front aspect of Sen Kalathari at the front of the shoulder. It does not match up with the Superficial Front Line at all. The erectors are part of the Superficial Back Line. The SBL strating at the plantar side of the feet the with the plantar fascia and the short toe flexors (Netter Plate 501) runs around and blends into the heel to turn and go straight up with the superficial posterior compartment of the lower leg, the Soleus and the Gastrocnemius (Netter Plate 485). This is a point where Kalathri has no match with the myofascial meridians, because it turns to the inside of the heel and runs at the inside of the legs.

Only if we go much further up we can rejoin with the SBL over the top of the hip where we can easily recognize the Erector spinae as the 2nd back line all the way to the occiput and to the Galea aponeurotica all the way to the eyebrows (Netter Plate 21).

This means there is a void on the back of the legs in the representation of Kalathari and I have a complex understanding of it. Kalathari turns from the front of the heel to the inside of the foot and the leg to form the 2nd inside energy line, which is really the medial edge of the Achilles tendon and the septum between Soleus and the Gastrocnemius. It probably does it in drawing on paper because Sen Sumana is already taking up the midline of the back side of the leg. But as I mentioned previously, Sen Sumana needs to be in the depth of the body not on the surface, therfore Kalathari can really be at the back of the leg connecting up to the hip with the hamstrings and to the erectors through the Sacrotuberous ligament (Netter Plate 465).

The last part of Sen Kalathari that needs to be clealrifyed is the criss-cross formation between shoulders and opposite hips and the 2nd inside line of the thigh also needs to be addressed. When I suggested that Sen Kalathari run up on the back of the legs I have omitted this part of the line.

This is where the Front Functional Line reveals itself. If we make a couple of exeptions of the Anatomy Train rules (the connection of the short head of the Biceps femoris and the extensors at the fibular head, and the fascial intervention of the Adductor magnus between the short head of the Biceps femoris and Adductor longus) we can find a connection from the tip of the toes to the head of the Fibula onto the Femur via the Short head of Biceps femoris and to the Adductor longus and all the way to the Pubic bone. Well, this extension of the Front Functional Line to the toes needs further validation.

It also means that the anterior medial intermuscular septum (Netter Plate 470) is the 2nd inside line of the thigh, and there we can find the emegence of the neuro-vascular bundle, that of course opens the access to perform the Blood stop (Exercise 2.8).

From here through the mechanical connections of the hip bones through the Pubic symphysis we can follow a sweep of continous fibers to the opposite side with the inner edge of the oblique fascia and to the outre edge of the Rectus abdominis. It is goes straight up to the 5th rib where links up with the lower edge of the Pectoralis major, which leads us to the Humerus (Netter Plate 174). The same pattern can be seen from the other side. I'll address the Arm Lines in a separate piece later. What is important to notice that the FFL doesn't play significant role in posture rather a big player in movement.

SEN SAHATSARANGSI (Left side of the body)
SEN THAWARI (right side of the body)

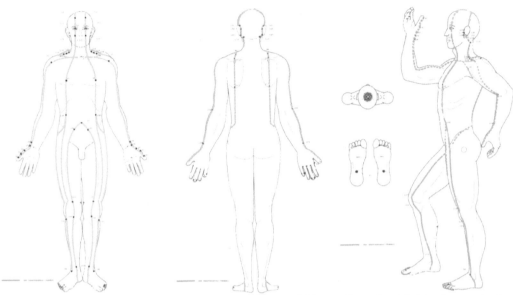

Illustration 15. Sen Sahatsarangsi-Thawari(Reproduced with kind permission from Andrea Baglioni)

Indications, therapy
Facial paralysis, toothache, throat ache, redness and swelling of the eye, fever, chest pain, maniac depression, gastrointestinal diseases, diseases of the urogenital system, leg paralysis, artrithis of the knee, numbness of the legs, hernia, knee pain

Tracing
Sen Sahatsarangi-Thawari run from the centre of the sole of the foot right front of the heel, around the foot towards the inside and the outside of the leg. The line continue on the inside of the lower legs as the 1st inside lines, and sharing the path with Sen Ittha/Pingkhala on the inner thigh. They move across the groin towards the abdomen in an arc to meet with Sen Sumana between the navel and the 2nd Chakra.

On the outside of the legs the lines run across the indentation between the foot and the leg in the centre of the dorsum of the foot and form the 1st outside lines on the legs. They split below the knees into two branches.

The top branch running right across the knees continuing in center of the thighs (this is an additional pathway to the 3 inside and 3 outside lines) and move onto the abdomen and into the kidney points of the abdomen.

From here the lines run towards the nipples, then to the throat and to the head to the centre of the eyes. Then they continue up on the head and turn towards the back of the ears. They circle around the ears and share the front of the ears with Sen Lawusang—Ulangka.

On the legs the other branch continue from the last point before the knees on the side of the knees and the thighs towards the boomerang but splits at the indentation just before the boomerang.

One aspect of the lines moving towards the abdomen, meeting the branch (the added pathway from accross the center of the thigh) at the kidney point where they terminate. The other aspect of the line crosses the boomerang halfway between the tip of the hip and the 3rd boomerang point, moving across the buttocks towards the back of the kidneys forming the 3rd backlines. The 3rd backlines cross the shoulder blades at the lowest tip of the scapulas moving up to the side of the neck and behind the ears.
At the front of the soft area on the shoulders the lines branch out towards the outside of the arms running towards the outside of the thumbs.

Below the collar bone the line branches out across the shoulders towards the inside of the arms and there inside the bone towards the side of the thumbs. The arm line towards the thumbs Sen Sanasarangsi-Thawari shares with Sen Sumana.

Exercises
Foot massage
1.4, 1.7, 1.8,
Lines on the leg
Palming and thumbing 1nd inside and outside lines on the legs in supine position
2.1-2.7
Single leg exercises
3.7, 3.9, 3.11, 3.16, 3-39
Front upper body
5.1, 5.2, 6.1, 7.1, 7.3, 7.4 hand massage thumb, 8.1
Side position
9.10, 9.11, 9.13, 9.19, 9.20, 9.22, 9.23, 9.24
Back position
10.8, 10.9, 10.10, 10.11
Sitting position
11.12

Spiral Line, Superficial Front Line – SL, SFL

Looking at Sen Sahatsarangsi-Thawari two features attract attention. One is the sling under the foot, and the other is the arch of the line below the navel that connects the insides of the two legs. These features point to the Spiral Line, and the main aspect of the legs of the Superficial Front Line of the Anatomy Trains to match with this set of Sen Lines. While these features are matching, there are details that make this correspondence feel like square pegs in round wholes.

The sling of the feet is a great match except the ugly fact that the Tibialis anterior connects the inside of the foot to the front and outside of the lower leg (1st outside line) and there isn't a myofascial unit that would connect the inside of the foot to the inside of the lower leg as the Thai Sen lines show. It is an issue caused by the human design that needs to be investigated in the future. Myofascially speaking the sling under the foot comprised of Tibialis anterior and Fibularis longus (together they are part of the Spiral Line) connection on the Medial cuneiform bone (Netter Plate 496), which means we shifted the sling to the anterior and lateral side of the leg from being anterior and medial.

Moving up on the legs Sen Sahatsarangsi-Thawari are taking the 1st lines on both inside and outside of the legs. If we follow Tibialis anterior instead of the 1st inside line, it takes us the patella through the Subpatellar tendon and onto the Rectus femoris (Netter Plate 488,462) which is the main aspect of the Superficial Front Line. This is the exact pathway of Sen Sahatsarangsi-Thawari on the thighs.
The origin of Rectus femoris is at the AIIS and that won't connect us to the upper part of the Spiral Line to the ASIS. Unless we make the same shift we suggested on the lower leg, from the anterior-medial to the anterior-lateral, and follow the anterior edge of the Iliotibial band and the TFL up to the Iliac crest and to the ASIS (Netter Plate 462). This change also needs further exploration as the SFL nicely fit with the characteristics and location of Sen Sahatsarangsi-Thawari.

It gets interesting when Sen Sahatsarangsi-Thawari move across the groin area. The Sen Lines coming from the outside of the leg continue straight up to the chest, while the lines that are coming from the inner legs join into each other below the navel.

It looks like the Spiral Line. Envision that these Sen Lines really crossing into each other, connecting the hips to the opposite shoulder or rather to the same side of the neck and Occiput, through the abdominal fascial continuations of the Internal oblique, external oblique through the rectus sheath (Netter Plate 232,233), to the Serratus anterior-Rhomboid unit that continues into the Splenius capitis muscle (Netter Plate 163,178). You may see this resemblance if you look at the body in 3 dimensionally and see the possible depth of these pathways.

Sen Sahatsarangsi-Thawari are very much represented on the front and underrepresented on the back side of the body, therefore it is missing from the comparison with the back side of the Spiral Line, which is the continuation of the long head of the Biceps femoris through the Sacrotuberous ligament and the erectors all the way up to the occiput. Even if we take a closer look at the back segments of Sen Sahatsarangsi-Thawari they really just pass over the scapulas. Can they mean the "rhombo-serratus" unit anterior to the Scapulas?

The other loop of Sen Sahatsarangsi-Thawari on the top of the head also brings the feeling that this set of Sen Lines really binding the energy body together. Similar to the SL that applies the same sling over the bottom of the feet and makes two crossings, one on the front over the abdomen and the other going under the scapulas and crossing over the spine to hook up the front and back side of the body at the occiput.

SEN LAWUSANG (left side of the body) SEN ULANGKA (Sen Rucham) (right side of the body)

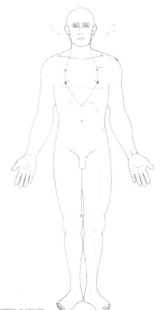

Illustration 16. Sen Lawusang-Ulangka(Reproduced with kind permission from Andrea Baglioni)

Indications, therapy
Deafness, ear diseases, middle ear infection, cough, facial paralysis, toothache, sore throat, chest pain, gastrointestinal diseases

Tracing
Sen Lawusang-Ulangka run from the solar plexus across me nipples towards the throat and to the front of the ear. They circle around the ears and share the back of the ears with Sen Sahatsarangshi-Thawari. From the front of the ears the lines move up the head and circle into Sen Sahatsarangsi-Thawari on the top of the head.

SEN NANTHAKRAVAT
Sen Nanthakrhavat runs as Sen Sikhini from the urethra to the navel and as Sen Sukhumang from the anus to the navel.

SEN KHITCHANNA
Sen Khitchanna runs from the penis as Sen Pitakun to the navel and as Sen Kitcha from the vagina to the navel.

The Arm Lines – SFAL, SBAL, DFAL, DBAL

We discuss the arm lines separate from the main aspects of the Sen Energy Lines because the pathways of the arms are shared, and because it is easier to show them paralell with the myofascial links. This is only chronological separation of course, both the Sen Energy Lines and the Anatomy Trains of the arms are seamlessly link up to the rest of the body.

The Sen Energy Line pathways of the arm are special. There are three lines inside and three lines on the outside of the arms, from the midline of the body –the sternum or the chakras- to the tip of the fingers. The 1st inside line shared by Sen Sumana and Ittha or Pingkhala, while the 3rd inside line shared by Sen Sumana and Sahatsarangsi or Thawari on the respective sides. Meanwhile Sen Kalathari takes the 2nd or center line by itself.

The back side or the outside of the arms are the same except Sen Sumana isn't presented. Sen Ittha and Pingkhala runs to the little finger on the 1st line, Sen Kalathari on the center again and Sen Sahatsarangsi Thawari on the thumb side takes the 3rd outside line.

Myofascially speaking there are four lines that are more or less equvivalent to the Sen Lines of the arms. Starting with the Superficial Front Arm Line, it is very easy to see Kalathari in it as it is passing the chest across with the fascia of the Pectoralis major –and unusually a back muscle, the anterior fibers of the Latissimus dorsi- into the center line of the arm, which is the medial intermuscular septum (Netter Plate 404,408,419). The SFAL then shoots toward the fingers with the flexor group through the Carpal tunnel to the Palmar surface of the fingers (Netter Plate 421,446). The very same pattern can be recognized on the outside of the arms in the SBAL. The wide spread Trapezius connects to the bundles of the Deltoid to link up with the Lateral intermuscular septum (Netter Plate 419) and the extensor group, to end at the dorsal surface of the fingers (Netter Plate 399,404,451).

Between the shared pathways on the inside of the arms only the thumb side has its own descrate myofascial link. It is the Deep Front Arm Line that starts with the Pectoralis minor to connect up with the Biceps Brachii via the Coracoid process (Netter Plate 408). From there the DFAL is linking down to the Thenar muscles through the Radial collateral ligaments (Netter Plate 412) to the outside of the thumb. It matches with Sen Sumana and Sen Sahatsarangsi-Thawari on the front of the arms but has very little in common on the back side of the arm with Sen Sahatsarangsi-Thawari.

On the outsdie of the arm we find the similar arrangment. Sen Ittha and Pingkhala clearly can be matched up with the Deep Back Arm Line (the Rhomboid muscle and Levator scapulae, the rotator cuff muscles, Triceps brachii, Ulnar periosteum, Ulnar collateral ligaments, Hypothenar muscles and the outside of the little finger (Netter Plate 407,412,420)) but very little resembelance on the front side for Sen Sumana and Sen Ittha-Pigkhala.

After all we can see how the Thai Sen Lines are surrounding the myofascial linkages on both, the little finger and the thumb sides from front and back. It is one of the major charactheristics of the Thai Energy theory that opens the door for further explorations.

Conclusion

To summarize all the above examined correspondance between the energy body and the physical body within the connective tissue, I'm still stunned that the two network are so much similar. The findings are these:

After I had the opportunity to work with Tom Myers and Todd Garcia a week long dissection I gained lot of inshight about the design of the human body. One of them was the 3 dimensional nature of our body. That made me think during writing this book and I recognized that all the Sen Lines are laid on the surface of the body and it looks alright on paper in a book. However in 3D with real bodies, depth and surface become really important. If we take a look at the Aura of a human, it always shown around us only on the coronal plane but really it is all over around us. Also come into my mind that different masters or traditions in Thai massage don't necessary agree on the pathways of the Sen Lines. Or when you look at a map of a geographic area you won't see the altitude of the mountains or hills and your trek may ends up twice as long as you have planned.

All of our knowledge about the Sen Lines comes from the carvings in the Wat Pho and from the practice handed over generations to generations. It is heavily secret knowledge and most of the massage schools or classes aren't giving clear information about the Sen Lines and their properties. I think going forward on this path and continue looking into the tracing and application of the Sen Lines we can enhance our healing art.

One such an interesting detail about the Sen Line Energy Line system that the side of the torso is not represented at all.

Other finding is that the Sen Lines are often located between muscle bundles or muscle groups. Working these openings between muscles with any kind of technique definitely increases the ability to slide on each other and makes the body more limber and freer.
Exploration of the arms lines, and the lines of the inner thigh shows that Sen lines tend to "surround" the myofascial units and it looks like the 2 dimensional nature of drawing causes this optical illusion. In the real 3 dimensional living body the Sen lines and the myofascial units are taking up space.

What we know is that Thai massage has always been a part of a bigger medical repertoar called Thai medicine, and never been a single remedy for any ailment. Therefore I can see Thai massage as the complementary and maintnance practice to Structural Integration to help create well needed energy, adaptability and segmentability. Also Thai massage should be used for energy balancing on regular base.

I learnt that in Thailand dissection isn't performed upon death for religious reasons, and that's why thai don't know about anatomy. During my research about Jivaka I have found out that Jivaka himself was a great surgeon with vast knowledge about the human body, probably due to bloody wars and fights where serious injuries were common. That makes me think that Thai massage have lost some of the original knowledge during the thousands of years.

After this initial comparison is about to be published, I'm looking forward to take the theory onto the mat within the Thai massage community and start playing around with the exercises to build supporting applications for receivers' postural needs.

Appendix

Structuring guide for the 2 hour Energy Balancing Thai yoga massage session by body types

Exercise No.	All	Stiff	MediumFlexible	Flexible	Description
Foot massage					Essential
1.1	■				Essential
1.2–1.6	■				
1.7	■				Choose one of the working order
1.8-1.12	■				
1.13					Optional
Energy lines of the leg					Essential Contraindication: varicose veins
2.1-2.7	■				Essential
2.8	■				Circulatory contraindications
Single leg exercises					
3.1-3.3		■			For stiff use pillow for MF and F choose one of them
3.4-3.9		■			
3.10	■				Essential
3.11			■	■	
3.12	■				Essential
3.13-3.15, 3.22	■				Optional for lower back and hamstrings
3.16-3.18	■				Optional for hamstrings and hip
3.19-3.20	■				Essential with variations
3.21	■				Contraindication for hernia
3.22			■	■	Optional
3.23 or 4.9	■				
3.24	■				
3.25.1-3.25.5	■				Essential with variations
3.26 or 9.21 or 9.24 or 11.8	■				3.26 for All 9.24 for F 11.8 not for Stiff 9.21 for Stiff
Double leg exercises					Contraindications: pregnancy, menstruation, high blood pressure, heart disease
4.1-4.2	■				
4.3			■	■	
4.4	■				
4.5	■				
4.6	■				
4.7			■	■	Not with serious lower back condition
4.8			■	■	
4.9			■	■	Contraindication: knee problem
4.10-4.12	■				Variations for bigger or smaller clients

Section					Description
Abdomen Massage					Contraindications: pregnancy, abdominal pain, full stomach leave 2 hours after meal,
5.1-5.3	■				Essential
Chest, arms, hands, and face massage					Contraindication: hypertension heart disease
6.1	■				Recommended
6.2-6.4	■				Essential
Arms and Hands					Essential
7.1-7.11	■				Essential
Head and face					Essential
8.1	■				Essential
Side Position					
9.1-9.2	■				Positioning
9.3-9.4.2	■				Essential
9.5-9.7	■				Optional
9.8-9.11	■				Essential
9.12-9.14	■				
9.15-9.16	■				Essential
9.17-9.18	■				
9.19-9.22.1	■				Essential
9.22.2-9.24			■	■	Optional
9.25	■				Essential
Back position					
10.1-10.2	■				Not for receivers with stiff ankle
10.3-10.4	■				Recommended
10.5	■				Essential
10.6	■				Optional
10.7	■				Essential
10.8-10.9			■	■	Choose one of them
10.10	■				Essential
10.11			■	■	Variations
10.12	■				
Sitting position					
11.1-11.9	■				
11.10-11.12			■	■	Optional
11.13-11.14	■				Essential

Relaxation exercises
PRANA EGG

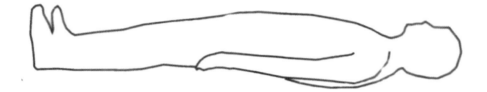

This exercise is based on 8:4 breathing rhythm.
Use your mind like a pencil. On the inhale, imagine drawing half of an oval beginning about 5 inches below your toes ending about 5 inches above your head on the right side of the body. On exhale, draw the other half of the egg on the left side of the body, starting at the head and down to the toes. You are lying now in the middle of a huge prana egg. Repeat the breathing and the visualization at least nine times.
This part of the exercise protects you from negative external energy influences.

Then start directly at the toes and on the in-breath draw the oval close to the body to the middle of the head, where the seventh chakra is situated.
On the exhale, close the egg on the left side from head to toes.
This part of the exercise creates self-confidence, equanimity and balance.
Repeat the breathing and the visualization at least nine times.

Form a small egg starting at the pelvis and ending at the 'third eye' the sixth Chakra. Visualize drawing the oval up on the right side on the inhale, down on the left side on the exhale. Repeat this part also at least nine times and you will be surrounded by an energy field allowing you deepest relaxation.

KAYA KRIYA

Kaya Kriya means 'body movement' and indeed, movement is an important part of this relaxation exercise.
In the starting position the legs are apart and the arms are spread away from the body. This exercise has four parts. Every part should be practiced at least eight to twelve times to ensure deep relaxation. If you do a more intensive practice, Kaya Kriya even helps to let go of grave psychic and physical tension.
Use 8:4 breathing rhythm.
In the first part of the exercise, control the breath into the lower part of the lungs and turn the feet and legs inward on the inhale. Apply as much pressure as possible. On the exhale, roll feet and legs outward again.
In the second part, breathe into the middle part of the lungs and roll arms and hands outward with strong pressure. Your back may slightly lift off the ground. Roll the arms and hands back inward on the exhale.

In the third part, breathe into the upper part of the lungs and turn the head to the right on the inhale, to the left on the exhale. In the fourth part, you do a full three-part breath and perform all three movements at the same time.

Then continue breath normally without any breathing control and maintain the relaxation posture for as long as you like often you can feel a tremendous energy play at this point. There is a powerful release of tension.

So whenever you feel really down and drained the Kaya Kriya may perform miracles. Take your time for this time-consuming exercise. It is worth it.

Starting
1 = inhalation
2 = exhalation

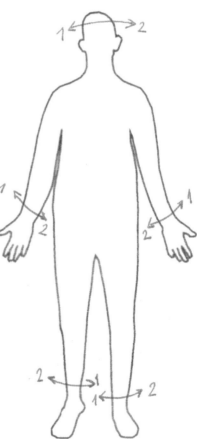

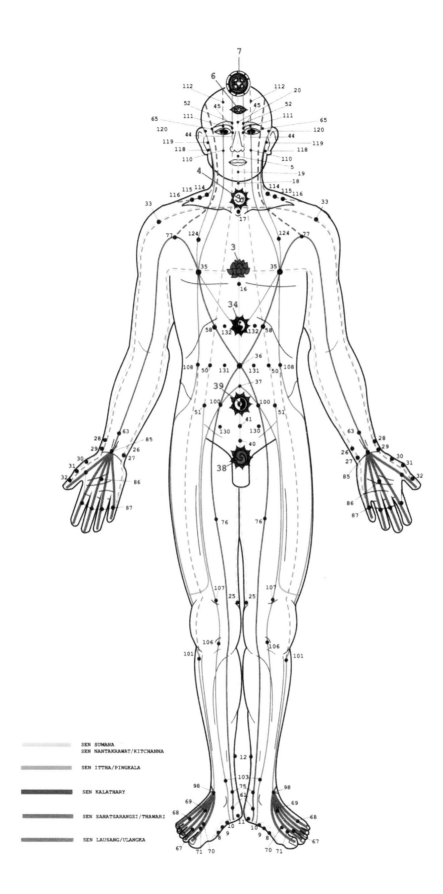

SEN SUMANA
SEN NANTAKRAWAT/KITCHANNA

SEN ITTHA/PINGKALA

SEN KALATHARY

SEN SAHATSARANGSI/THAWARI

SEN LAUSANG/ULANGKA

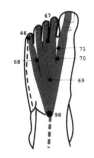

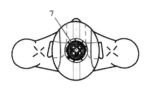

7

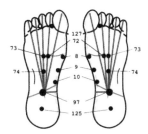

67
46
68
71
70
69
98

127
72
73   73
8
74   74
9
10
97
125

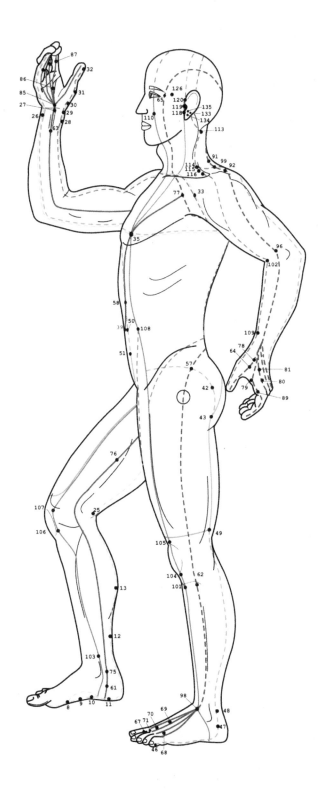

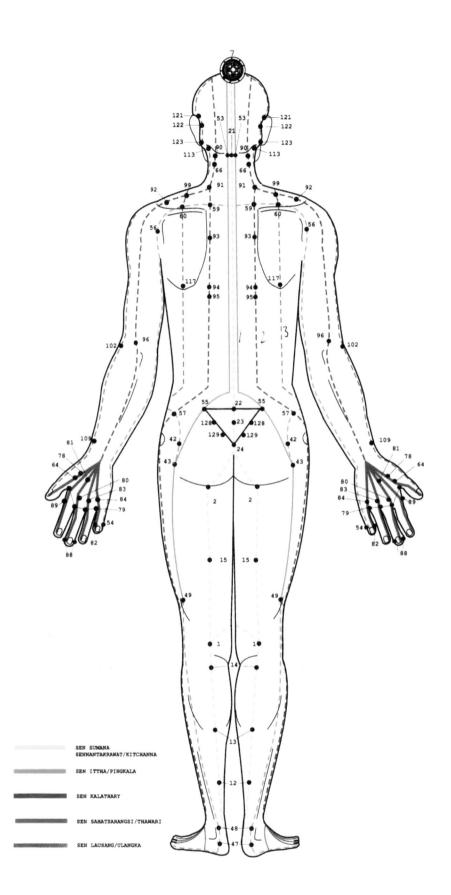

SEN SUMANA
SENNANTAKRAWAT/KITCHANNA

SEN ITTHA/PINGKALA

SEN KALATHARY

SEN SAHATSARANGSI/THAWARI

SEN LAUSANG/ULANGKA

Bibliography

Encyclopaedic dictionary of the Dharmaśāstra By Swami Parmeshwaranand, Sarup, 2003, 542 p

History of medicine in India: the medical encounter By Chittabrata Palit, Achintya Kumar Dutta

C. Pierce Salguero, The History of Traditional Thai Medicine Reconsidered Asokananda(Harald Brust), The Art of Traditional Thai Massage, DK Editions Duang Kamol, 1990 10th edition 2004

Asokananda(Harald Brust), The Art of Traditional Thai Massage Energy Line Charts, DK Editions Duang Kamol, 1990, 2nd edition 2001

Asokananda(Harald Brust), The Art of Traditional Thai Massage in the Side Position, DK Editions Duang Kamol, 2001

Asokananda(Harald Brust), Thus Have I Heard, Nai Suk's Editions Cxo. Ltd. 1994, 1999

Richard Gold , Thai Massage A traditional Medical Technique, 2nd edition, Mosby Elsevier 2007

Chongkol Setthakorn, Sen-Therapy Nuad Bo Rarn Ancient massage of Thailand

Andrea Baglioni, Lower back, shoulder and Neck Therapies - Manual

Kaczvinszky József, Kelet világossága, Kötet Kiadó, 1995

Sivananda yoga Vedanta center, Yoga Mind&Body, DK Publishing Inc. 1996

Thomas Myers, Body3

Thomas W. Myers, AnatomyTrains Elsevier Science Limited, 2001

Frank H. Netter, Atlas of Human Anatomy, Ciba-Geigy Corporation, 1989

Rosemary Feitis, Ida Rolf Talks About Rolfing and Physical Reality, Harper & Row, 1978

Made in the USA
Lexington, KY
17 July 2010